Features of Pathogenesis of Human Viral Infections and Antiviral Drugs

Features of Pathogenesis of Human Viral Infections and Antiviral Drugs

Editor

Stefano Aquaro

MDPI • Basel • Beijing • Wuhan • Barcelona • Belgrade • Manchester • Tokyo • Cluj • Tianjin

Editor
Stefano Aquaro
Department of Pharmacy,
Health, and Nutritional Sciences,
University of Calabria
Italy

Editorial Office
MDPI
St. Alban-Anlage 66
4052 Basel, Switzerland

This is a reprint of articles from the Special Issue published online in the open access journal *Medicina* (ISSN 1010-660X) (available at: https://www.mdpi.com/journal/medicina/special_issues/human_viral_infections).

For citation purposes, cite each article independently as indicated on the article page online and as indicated below:

LastName, A.A.; LastName, B.B.; LastName, C.C. Article Title. *Journal Name* **Year**, *Volume Number*, Page Range.

ISBN 978-3-03943-917-1 (Hbk)
ISBN 978-3-03943-918-8 (PDF)

Contents

About the Editor vii

Preface to "Features of Pathogenesis of Human Viral Infections and Antiviral Drugs" ix

Cristina Iulia Mitran, Ilinca Nicolae, Mircea Tampa, Madalina Irina Mitran, Constantin Caruntu, Maria Isabela Sarbu, Corina Daniela Ene, Clara Matei, Antoniu Cringu Ionescu, Simona Roxana Georgescu and Mircea Ioan Popa
The Relationship between the Soluble Receptor for Advanced Glycation End Products and Oxidative Stress in Patients with Palmoplantar Warts
Reprinted from: *Medicina* **2019**, *55*, 706, doi:10.3390/medicina55100706 1

Essam M. Janahi, Zahra Ilyas, Sara Al-Othman, Abdulla Darwish, Sanad J. Sanad, Budoor Almusaifer, Mariam Al-Mannai, Jamal Golbahar and Simone Perna
Hepatitis B Virus Genotypes in the Kingdom of Bahrain: Prevalence, Gender Distribution and Impact on Hepatic Biomarkers
Reprinted from: *Medicina* **2019**, *55*, 622, doi:10.3390/medicina55100622 11

Liubov Biliavska, Yulia Pankivska, Olga Povnitsa and Svitlana Zagorodnya
Antiviral Activity of Exopolysaccharides Produced by Lactic Acid Bacteria of the Genera *Pediococcus*, *Leuconostoc* and *Lactobacillus* against Human Adenovirus Type 5
Reprinted from: *Medicina* **2019**, *55*, 519, doi:10.3390/medicina55090519 21

Raffaele Del Prete, Luigi Ronga, Grazia Addati, Raffaella Magrone, Angela Abbasciano, Domenico Di Carlo and Luigi Santacroce
A Retrospective Study about the Impact of Switching from Nested PCR to Multiplex Real-Time PCR on the Distribution of the Human Papillomavirus (HPV) Genotypes
Reprinted from: *Medicina* **2019**, *55*, 418, doi:10.3390/medicina55080418 33

Ana Borrajo, Alessandro Ranazzi, Michela Pollicita, Maria Concetta Bellocchi, Romina Salpini, Maria Vittoria Mauro, Francesca Ceccherini-Silberstein, Carlo Federico Perno, Valentina Svicher and Stefano Aquaro
Different Patterns of HIV-1 Replication in MACROPHAGES is Led by Co-Receptor Usage
Reprinted from: *Medicina* **2019**, *55*, 297, doi:10.3390/medicina55060297 43

Daifullah Al Aboud, Nora M. Al Aboud, Mater I. R. Al-Malky and Ahmed S. Abdel-Moneim
Genotyping of Type A Human Respiratory Syncytial Virus Based on Direct F Gene Sequencing
Reprinted from: *Medicina* **2019**, *55*, 169, doi:10.3390/medicina55050169 61

About the Editor

Stefano Aquaro is a full professor of Microbiology and Clinical Microbiology as well as a full professor of Virology at the University of Calabria, Italy (2006–present), where he is also the head of Microbiology and Virology Laboratory Dept. of Pharmacy, Health and Nutritional Sciences. He is an M.D. graduated with full marks at University of Rome "Tor Vergata", Italy, and a consultant in Medical Microbiology and Virology (University of Rome "Tor Vergata" cum Laude). He was also the head of the "Home Care Unit for people living with HIV/AIDS in Rome", NPO, Italy (1994–1996). He was equally the founder and president of R.O.M.A. (Research Office and Medical Assistance) NPO, providing home care for people living with HIV/AIDS and chronic diseases (2000–2005). Furthermore, Professor Aquaro was a research fellow at the Dept. of Experimental Medicine and Biochemical Sciences, University of Rome "Tor Vergata", Italy (1995–1999). He has also been an associate research professor of Virology at the Faculty of Medicine, University of Rome "Tor Vergata", Italy (1999–2002). He has also been a researcher (1999–2001) and a visiting professor (October–December 2004) at the Laboratory of Virology and Chemotherapy, "Rega Institute", Catholic University of Leuven, Belgium. He was also a research professor at the Dept. of Experimental Medicine and Biochemical Sciences, University of Rome "Tor Vergata", Italy (2002–2006), and a member of the Committee, School of Doctorate in Medical Microbiology and Immunology, University of Rome "Tor Vergata", Italy (2003–2006). Finally, he has been a member of the Committee, School of Doctorate in Cellular Biochemistry and drugs activity in Oncology, University of Calabria, Italy (2007–2012), as well as of the Committee, School of Doctorate in Translational medicine, University of Calabria, Italy (2013–present). His research is mainly focused on virus evolution, virus virulence and pathogenicity, and antiviral drugs.

Preface to "Features of Pathogenesis of Human Viral Infections and Antiviral Drugs"

Among infectious diseases, viral infections are the leading cause of death worldwide, especially in the most low-income countries, particularly in young children. Most of the human viruses are all well characterized in terms of structure, life-cycle, tropism, and associated primary pathologies, but many of the pathogenetic mechanisms underlying their ability to cause acute infection, persist or reactivate in the host and cause chronic and/or degenerative damage, and still need to be fully clarified. At the same time, it seems necessary to develop novel therapeutic approaches and rationale, and possibly more potent antiviral compounds that are addressed to novel targets.

Stefano Aquaro
Editor

medicina

MDPI

Article

The Relationship between the Soluble Receptor for Advanced Glycation End Products and Oxidative Stress in Patients with Palmoplantar Warts

Cristina Iulia Mitran [1,2], Ilinca Nicolae [3], Mircea Tampa [1,3,*], Madalina Irina Mitran [1,2], Constantin Caruntu [1,4,*], Maria Isabela Sarbu [1], Corina Daniela Ene [5], Clara Matei [1], Antoniu Cringu Ionescu [1], Simona Roxana Georgescu [1,3,*] and Mircea Ioan Popa [1,2]

1 "Carol Davila" University of Medicine and Pharmacy, 020021 Bucharest, Romania; cristina.iulia.mitran@gmail.com (C.I.M.); madalina.irina.mitran@gmail.com (M.I.M.); isabela_sarbu@yahoo.com (M.I.S.); matei_clara@yahoo.com (C.M.); antoniuginec@yahoo.com (A.C.I.); mircea.ioan.popa@gmail.com (M.I.P.)

2 "Cantacuzino" National Medico-Military Institute for Research and Development, 011233 Bucharest, Romania

3 "Victor Babes" Clinical Hospital for Infectious Diseases, 030303 Bucharest, Romania; drnicolaei@yahoo.ro

4 "Prof. N. Paulescu" National Institute of Diabetes, Nutrition and Metabolic Diseases, 011233 Bucharest, Romania

5 "Carol Davila' Nephrology Hospital", 010731 Bucharest, Romania; koranik85@yahoo.com

* Correspondence: dermatology.mt@gmail.com (M.T.); costin.caruntu@gmail.com (C.C.); srg.dermatology@gmail.com (S.R.G.)

Received: 28 August 2019; Accepted: 16 October 2019; Published: 20 October 2019

Abstract: *Background and objectives*: Warts are the most common lesions caused by human papillomavirus (HPV). Recent research suggests that oxidative stress and inflammation are involved in the pathogenesis of HPV-related lesions. It has been shown that the soluble receptor for advanced glycation end products (sRAGE) may act as a protective factor against the deleterious effects of inflammation and oxidative stress, two interconnected processes. However, in HPV infection, the role of sRAGE, constitutively expressed in the skin, has not been investigated in previous studies. *Materials and Methods*: In order to analyze the role of sRAGE in warts, we investigated the link between sRAGE and the inflammatory response on one hand, and the relationship between sRAGE and the total oxidant/antioxidant status (TOS/TAS) on the other hand, in both patients with palmoplantar warts (n = 24) and healthy subjects as controls (n = 28). *Results*: Compared to the control group, our results showed that patients with warts had lower levels of sRAGE (1036.50 ± 207.60 pg/mL vs. 1215.32 ± 266.12 pg/mL, $p < 0.05$), higher serum levels of TOS (3.17 ± 0.27 vs. 2.93 ± 0.22 µmol H2O2 Eq/L, $p < 0.01$), lower serum levels of TAS (1.85 ± 0.12 vs. 2.03 ± 0.14 µmol Trolox Eq/L, $p < 0.01$) and minor variations of the inflammation parameters (high sensitivity-CRP, interleukin-6, fibrinogen, and erythrocyte sedimentation rate). Moreover, in patients with warts, sRAGE positively correlated with TAS (r = 0.43, $p < 0.05$), negatively correlated with TOS (r = −0.90, $p < 0.01$), and there was no significant correlation with inflammation parameters. There were no significant differences regarding the studied parameters between groups when we stratified the patients according to the number of the lesions and disease duration. *Conclusions*: Our results suggest that sRAGE acts as a negative regulator of oxidative stress and could represent a mediator involved in the development of warts. However, we consider that the level of sRAGE cannot be used as a biomarker for the severity of warts. To the best of our knowledge, this is the first study to demonstrate that sRAGE could be involved in HPV pathogenesis and represent a marker of oxidative stress in patients with warts.

Keywords: sRAGE; oxidative stress; inflammation; warts; HPV

1. Introduction

Warts are muco-cutaneous lesions caused by human papillomavirus (HPV) [1]. Warts are very common in the general population, with up to one third of the children being affected; the incidence decreases with age. Considering that immunity plays an important role in the development of warts, the incidence increases up to 45% among immunosuppressed individuals [2]. To this date, more than 200 HPV types have been identified [3]. Warts are commonly associated with HPV 1, 2, 4 and 7. In immunosuppressed patients, HPV 75, 76 and 77 were identified. Warts manifest as skin-colored papules with a keratotic surface. Most frequently, the lesions involve the hands and feet, but they can also appear on extension areas (elbows, knees) [4,5]. Transmission of the infection occurs through direct contact in the context of skin microlesions or more rarely, indirectly through contaminated objects [5]. The incubation period ranges from 1 to 20 months; there is no systemic spread of the virus. HPV infects host cells without integrating viral DNA into their genome [6].

Warts occur when HPV infects the upper layers of the skin or mucous membranes, resulting in abnormal and rapid cell growth. There are several conditions that contribute to the acquisition of HPV infection, including incomplete immune system development, CD4+ T-cell dysfunction, other causes of immunosuppression, and the alteration of the normal epithelial barrier [7–13]. Most often in children, warts resolve spontaneously, without treatment, but the lesions can be persistent in adults. However, recurrences are common in both groups [10,11]. There is no clear evidence of the etiopathogenic mechanisms of HPV infection. Multiple factors contributing to its pathogenesis have been suggested, such as the lack of efficient protective cell mechanisms against the virus and the accumulation of toxic compounds which induce oxidative stress and inflammation [14–19]. Oxidative stress and inflammation are two interconnected processes which produce multiple effects on cell function [20].

The 45 kDa receptor for advanced glycation end products (RAGE) is a member of the immunoglobulin superfamily, which contains an extracellular region of 320 amino acids (sequence 23–342), a 21-amino acid transmembrane hydrophobic region (sequence 343–363) and a cytoplasmic region of 41 amino acids (sequence 364–404). The extracellular region is composed of two C-type domains (C1 consisting of 124–221 amino acid residues and C2 consisting of 227–317 amino acid residues) and a V-type domain (sequence 23–116 amino acid residues). The V domain confers the ability to bind various ligands. The V and C1 domains are involved in the stability/specificity of the receptor-ligand complex. The C2 domain participates in the dimerization/oligomerization of receptor-ligand complexes. The receptor is anchored to the cell membrane through its transmembrane domain. The endocellular domain is essential for intracellular signaling [21–23].

Many studies have shown that RAGE has a large number of ligands, such as advanced glycation end products (AGEs), S100 calgranulin proteins, high motility group box 1 protein, amyloid fibrils, phosphatidylserine, macrophage-1 antigen, lipopolysaccharide from the outer membrane of Gram-negative bacteria, peptidoglycan (present in the majority of bacteria), lipoteichoic acid (a component of many Gram-positive bacteria), bacterial DNA, viral DNA/RNA, yeast cell wall mannans, degraded extracellular matrix components, and modified fibronectin [15,18,24,25].

RAGE has been found during embryonic development, its expression being reduced in adulthood, excepting the lung and skin [17]. Other cells, such as monocytes/macrophages, smooth muscle cells, endothelial cells, fibroblasts, and neuronal cells, do not express physiologically detectable amounts, but receptor expression may be induced during cell stress in various instances including the accumulation of the ligands of RAGE, or when the transcriptional factors which modulate the expression of RAGE are activated [26,27]. Soluble RAGE (sRAGE) acts as a decoy for RAGE ligands, preventing their interactions with membrane RAGE (mRAGE) through a competitive mechanism, and consequently, sRAGE disrupts the generation of oxidative stress and inflammation [14]. Increased amounts of RAGE ligands induce the overexpression of sRAGE [27].

To the best of our knowledge, the role of sRAGE in the onset and progression of warts has not been previously investigated. To analyze the possible molecular mechanisms involved in the development of cutaneous warts, we hypothesized that sRAGE acts as an endogenous factor able to maintain/restore the cutaneous homeostasis. We have analyzed the interaction between circulating sRAGE and inflammatory response on the one hand and the relationship between sRAGE and oxidant/antioxidant status on the other hand in patients with palmoplantar warts (Figure 1).

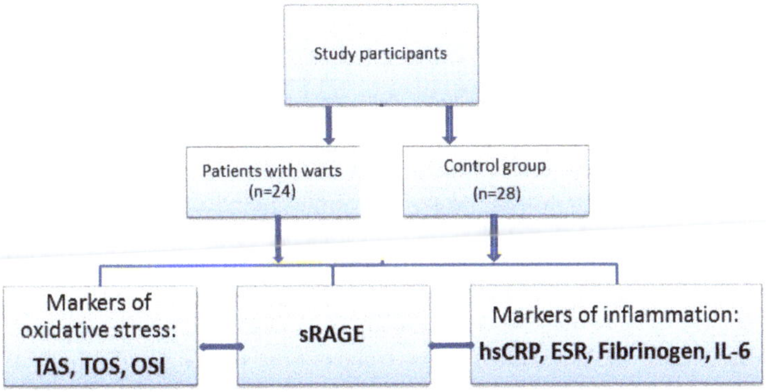

Figure 1. The plan of investigation of sRAGE in association with oxidative stress and inflammation in patients with warts. sRAGE = soluble receptor for advanced glycation end products, TAS = total antioxidant status, TOS = total oxidant status, OSI = oxidative stress index, ESR = erythrocyte sedimentation rate, hs-CRP = high-sensitive C reactive protein, Il-6 = interleukin-6.

2. Materials and Methods

2.1. Study Participants

The patients were selected from those who presented to the Clinic of Dermatology and were diagnosed with palmoplantar warts, the most common HPV-related lesions. All study participants gave their consent to the use of their biological samples in research studies. All the procedures and the experiments performed in the study respect the ethical standards in the Helsinki Declaration, as well as the national law. The study protocol was approved by the Ethics Committee of "Victor Babes Infectious and Tropical Diseases Hospital" (13050/31.07.2017).

Inclusion criteria: otherwise healthy adults, aged 18 years or above; adequate nutritional status; non-smokers; and with no treatment for warts.

Exclusion criteria from the study (conditions widely known as being able to alter, and therefore interfere with parameters of inflammation and oxidative stress): chronic alcohol use, drug abuse; treatment with corticosteroids, immunosuppressant agents and nutritional supplements; and pregnancy and breastfeeding.

Based on similar demographic characteristics, the study participants were divided into two groups: patients with palmoplantar warts ($n = 24$) and healthy subjects as controls ($n = 28$). We analyzed the serum levels of sRAGE, oxidative stress parameters and markers of inflammation compared to controls. We also evaluated the levels of sRAGE, oxidative stress parameters and markers of inflammation according to the number of the lesions and the duration of the disease. According to the number of the lesions we stratified the patients into three groups: less than 5 lesions ($n = 11$), between 5–10 lesions ($n = 8$) and more than 10 lesions ($n = 5$). The distribution of the patients with warts according to the duration of the disease divided them into three groups: with a history of less than 1 month ($n = 6$), between 1 and 6 months ($n = 10$) and a history longer than 6 months ($n = 8$).

2.2. Laboratory Tests

Biological samples were drawn from the patients and controls enrolled in the study under basal conditions using a holder-vacutainer system. Venous blood collected on anticoagulant (K3EDTA) was used to determine the blood count and erythrocyte sedimentation rate. The samples were processed immediately. The plasma obtained from venous blood collected on heparin was used for serum fibrinogen determination. Serum was obtained from venous blood collected in vacutainer without anticoagulant. The hemolyzed or lactescent samples were rejected.

sRAGE levels were measured by ELISA method; the sandwich variant and the results were expressed as pg/mL. In the wells of a polystyrene plate in which known antibodies were attached, the unknown antigen solution was added and then incubated. After washing, enzyme-labelled antibodies were added and fixed to the free epitopes of a polyvalent antigen. After incubation, the wells were washed again. The presence of the labelled complex was detected using a chromogenic substrate (BioVision reagents, TECAN analyzer). The absorbance of the resulted yellow product was measured. The intensity of the color of the resulted product is proportional to the amount of sRAGE in the sample. To determine the concentrations of sRAGE in the samples, a standard curve was used. The intensity of the color was measured at 450 nm.

The following parameters were used to assess oxidative stress: total antioxidant status (TAS), total oxidant status (TOS), and oxidative stress index (OSI).

TOS and TAS levels were determined by spectrophotometric method (Randox reagents, HumaStar 300 analyzer); results were expressed as μmol of H_2O_2 equivalent/L serum for TOS and as μmol Trolox equivalent/L serum for TAS. OSI value was calculated using the following formula:

$$\text{OSI (arbitrary units)} = \frac{\text{TOS}\left(\mu\text{mol } H_2O_2\text{Eq}/\text{L}\right)}{\text{TAS}\left(\mu\text{mol Trolox Eq}/\text{L}\right)} \quad (1)$$

For the early detection of inflammation, the following determinations were used: high sensitivity C-reactive protein (hs-CRP, latex-immunoturbidimetric method), interleukin-6 (IL-6, ELISA method, sandwich variant, automatic reading method), the erythrocyte sedimentation rate (ESR, automatic reading method), and fibrinogen (coagulometric method).

2.3. *Statistical Analysis*

The comparison of obtained experimental data between groups was carried out using t-test. When we compared more than 2 groups we used Kruskal-Wallis test. The relationship between pairs of two parameters was assessed by Spearman's correlation coefficient after adequate assessment of normality of data using Kolmogorov-Smirnov test. We chose a significance level (p) of 0.05 (5%) and a confidence interval of 95% for hypothesis testing.

3. Results

The mean serum levels of sRAGE were significantly lower in patients with warts compared to healthy controls (1036.50 ± 207.60 pg/mL vs. 1215.32 ± 266.12 pg/mL, $p < 0.05$) (Table 1). Differences were also obtained for TAS levels (1.85 ± 0.12 vs. 2.03 ± 0.14 μmol Trolox Eq/L, $p < 0.05$), TOS levels (3.17 ± 0.27 vs. 2.93 ± 0.22 μmol H_2O_2 Eq/L, $p < 0.01$) and OSI (1.72 ± 0.22 vs. 1.45 ± 0.17, $p < 0.01$) compared to controls, (Table 1). The determination of the markers of inflammation did not reveal a relevant inflammatory process in patients with warts. The only exception was represented by hs-CRP levels. The mean level of hs-CRP was 0.19 ± 0.14 mg/dL in patients with warts and 0.06 ± 0.02 mg/dL in controls ($p < 0.05$). In contrast, IL-6, fibrinogen, and ESR did not show significant differences between the two groups (Table 1).

Table 1. The serum levels of sRAGE, oxidative stress parameters and markers of inflammation in patients with warts versus controls (expressed as mean and standard deviation).

Parameter	Patients with Warts n = 24	Controls n = 28	p Value
sRAGE (pg/mL)	1036.50 ± 207.60	1215.32 ± 266.12	<0.05 *
Markers of oxidative stress			
TAS (μmol Trolox Eq/L).	1.85 ± 0.12	2.03 ± 0.14	<0.01 *
TOS (μmol H_2O_2 Eq/L)	3.17 ± 0.27	2.93 ± 0.22	<0.01 *
OSI (arbitrary units)	1.72 ± 0.22	1.45 ± 0.17	<0.01 *
Markers of inflammation			
hs-CRP (mg/dL)	0.19 ± 0.14	0.06 ± 0.02	<0.01 *
ESR (mm/h)	5.20 ± 3.30	3.80 ± 2.10	>0.05
Fibrinogen (mg/dL)	183.5 ± 59.10	179.6 ± 64.70	>0.05
IL-6 (pg/mL)	7.62 ± 2.60	7.00 ± 2.40	>0.05

n = number of the patients. *—statistically significant.

The serum levels of the studied parameters did not differ significantly according to the number of the lesions between the groups (Table 2).

Table 2. The serum levels of sRAGE, oxidative stress parameters and markers of inflammation in patients with warts (expressed as mean and standard deviation) according to the number of the lesions.

Parameter	Patients with Warts <5 (n = 11)	Patients with Warts 5–10 (n = 8)	Patients with Warts >10 (n = 5)	p Value
sRAGE (pg/mL)	1029.45 ± 237.52	10,562.5 ± 204.47	1020.4 ± 179.90	0.9
Markers of oxidative stress				
TAS (μmol Trolox Eq/L).	1.83 ± 0.12	1.85 ± 0.11	1.89 ± 0.17	0.58
TOS (μmol H_2O_2 Eq/L)	3.23 ± 0.35	3.10 ± 0.21	3.17 ± 0.24	0.62
OSI (arbitrary units)	1.77 ± 0.23	1.68 ± 0.15	1.70 ± 0.30	0.52
Markers of inflammation				
hs-CRP (mg/dL)	0.19 ± 0.16	0.20 ± 0.16	0.19 ± 0.11	0.9
ESR (mm/h)	6.00 ± 3.58	4.50 ± 3.11	4.60 ± 3.13	0.8
Fibrinogen (mg/dL)	171.72 ± 53.20	191.37 ± 57.58	206.4 ± 78.00	0.6
IL-6 (pg/mL)	7.93 ± 2.72	7.49 ± 2.63	7.16 ± 2.93	0.9

The patients were divided into three groups; n = number of the patients.

There were no significantly differences between groups when we stratified patients according to the duration of the disease (Table 3).

Table 3. The serum levels of sRAGE, oxidative stress parameters and markers of inflammation in patients with warts (expressed as mean and standard deviation) according to the duration of the disease (months).

Parameter	Patients with Warts <1 (n = 6)	Patients with Warts 1–6 (n = 10)	Patients with Warts >6 (n = 8)	p Value
sRAGE (pg/mL)	1061.00 ± 278.63	1090.50 ± 207.13	950.62 ± 133.72	0.26
Markers of oxidative stress				
TAS (μmol Trolox Eq/L).	1.86 ± 0.12	1.88 ± 0.14	1.82 ± 0.12	0.49
TOS (μmol H_2O_2 Eq/L)	3.13 ± 0.20	3.16 ± 0.33	3.22 ± 0.30	0.91
OSI (arbitrary units)	1.69 ± 0.10	1.70 ± 0.27	1.78 ± 0.22	0.79
Markers of inflammation				
hs-CRP (mg/dL)	0.20 ± 0.13	0.21 ± 0.16	0.19 ± 0.16	0.82
ESR (mm/h)	7.17 ± 3.87	4.00 ± 2.45	5.25 ± 3.41	0.23
Fibrinogen (mg/dL)	182.33 ± 67.45	185.20 ± 55.23	188.25 ± 65.53	0.87
IL-6 (pg/mL)	6.92 ± 3.16	8.12 ± 2.24	7.53 ± 2.89	0.92

The patients were divided into three groups; n = number of the patients.

In patients with warts, sRAGE levels showed a positive statistically significant association with TAS (rho = 0.43, $p < 0.05$) and a negative statistically significant association with both TOS (rho = −0.90, $p < 0.01$) and OSI (rho = −0.86, $p < 0.01$) (Table 3). There was a lack of correlation between the levels of sRAGE and hs-CRP, IL-6, fibrinogen, and ESR in patients with warts (Table 4).

Table 4. The relationship between sRAGE and the markers of oxidative stress and inflammation, in patients with warts.

Parameter	Rho	*p* Value
TAS	0.43	<0.05 *
TOS	−0.90	<0.01 *
OSI	−0.86	<0.01 *
hs-CRP	0.11	>0.05
ESR	−0.10	>0.05
Fibrinogen	0.04	>0.05
IL-6	−0.14	>0.05

*—statistically significant.

4. Discussion

The serum concentration of sRAGE seems to be modulated by a complex group of factors such as genetic factors, internal and environmental stimuli [27–33]. It has also been suggested that serum levels of sRAGE are influenced by gender, age, ethnicity, the imbalance between antioxidants and prooxidants and inflammatory processes [27]. There are studies which attribute to sRAGE the role of a potential biomarker of oxidative stress [34]. Some reports have suggested that the overexpression of sRAGE reflects the excessive inflammatory response involved in the progression of endothelial lesions and coagulopathy associated with severe infection. Low levels of sRAGE were associated with increased levels of IL-6, VCAM-1 and PAI-1 as well as with thrombocytopenia [35]. At the same time, in patients with type 1 diabetes, sRAGE overexpression in response to increased levels of AGEs was interpreted as a modality of protection against cell damage. Under these conditions, sRAGE acts as a negative feedback mediator for eliminating AGEs. The overexpression of sRAGE can be considered a weapon against cell damage and a mechanism to regulate the receptor synthesis by modulating the synthesis of enzymes that produce a proteolytic cleavage [36].

In our study, we have found that patients with palmoplantar warts had lower serum levels of sRAGE compared to controls. sRAGE downregulation may be a factor involved in HPV pathogenesis; it can be speculated that sRAGE acts as a negative regulator of warts occurrence and could represent an early mediator involved in the onset and development of warts. The decrease in sRAGE levels in patients with palmoplantar warts could be explained by different mechanisms. HPV induces increased proliferation of keratinocytes resulting in a higher rate of glucose metabolism in the infected cells, which stimulates the synthesis of AGEs. Thus, AGEs accumulate in extracellular spaces and interact with sRAGE [37]. Another possible explanation is the disruption of the AGEs-sRAGE axis that might induce a low synthesis of soluble receptors [18,36,38]. sRAGE is cleaved on cell surface through the action of matrix metalloproteinases. The activity of these enzymes is modulated by oxidized lipoproteins [32]. It has also been reported that advanced glycosylation of high density lipoproteins leads to endogenous sRAGE sequestration [32,33].

The relationship between RAGE expression in the skin and the level of its ligands remains unclear. In human skin, sRAGE was positively correlated with the expression of genes encoding for ligands of RAGE such as tumor necrosis factor (TNF) alpha, IL-1 alpha, S100B, proapoptotic factors (Fas, Bax), epidermal differentiation markers (involucrin), and proliferating cell nuclear antigen [17]. Another factor that could influence sRAGE activity is the presence of a group of cell surface receptors, AGE-R1, AGE-R2, and AGE-R3, which seem to modulate the endocytosis and degradation of AGEs, thus counteracting the effects of RAGE. AGE-R1 has been shown to reduce oxidative stress induced by AGEs through the inhibition of RAGE signaling pathway [37].

Another point analyzed in our study was the investigation of potential mechanisms by which sRAGE is involved in the pathogenesis of warts. To demonstrate this hypothesis, we have performed a complete, simultaneous and comparable analysis of the axis sRAGE – markers of oxidative stress – markers of inflammation in patients with warts and in a control group. First, we have investigated oxidative stress markers (TOS, TAS, OSI) and confirmed the presence of an imbalance between oxidant load and antioxidant defense in patients with warts. Previous studies have suggested that the balance between oxidants and antioxidants plays an important role in the spontaneous regression of HPV infection, and the antioxidant system prevents the effects of oxidative stress and mediates the immune response [39,40]. A recent study has shown that oxidative stress plays an important role in recalcitrant warts [41]. Excessive amounts of oxidants lead to destructive effects, materialized in the structural and functional alteration of lipids, proteins and nucleotides [42]. In this case, the antioxidant systems may become deficient, favoring the perpetuation of oxidative stress. We consider that sRAGE can participate in the restoration of the oxidant/antioxidant balance in patients with warts. This hypothesis is supported by the strong negative correlation between sRAGE and TOS, respectively OSI, and the positive association between sRAGE and TAS. Based on these results, we assign to sRAGE the role of a potential biomarker of oxidative stress in patients with warts. Therefore, the modulation of sRAGE level in HPV patients might influence the progression of the disease.

In our study, the evaluation of a panel of markers of inflammation did not reveal an inflammatory systemic process in patients with warts. The sRAGE level was not correlated with the levels of the markers of inflammation (IL-6, fibrinogen and ESR) excepting hs-CRP. However, we do not exclude the presence of a proinflammatory environment in infected tissues. The association between sRAGE and hs-CRP has also been proven in several pathological conditions [43]. CRP is synthesized by hepatocytes in response to TNF alpha, IL-1, and IL-6 [44]. The AGEs-RAGE interaction increases the expression of these cytokines; sRAGE and RAGE compete for the same ligands. As a result, low sRAGE levels increase the AGEs-mRAGE interaction, which leads to increased cytokine production. It is known that sRAGE modulates the synthesis of hs-CRP in patients with acute coronary syndrome [45].

We have identified that none of the examined parameters was influenced by the extension of warts and disease duration. Our results are in concordance with the study by Sasmaz et al., which has also revealed that markers of oxidative stress (catalase, glucose-6-phosphate dehydrogenase, superoxide dismutase, and malondialdehyde) did not correlate with the duration and the number of the lesions [46]. We consider that the level of sRAGE cannot be used as a biomarker for the severity of warts. The molecular mechanisms by which sRAGE could be involved in the etiopathogenesis of warts are complex and could include the interference between oxidative stress and inflammation.

In our study, we have shown changes of serum levels of sRAGE in patients with palmoplantar warts compared to the control group. Given that warts are produced by HPV we have suggested a possible role of sRAGE in the pathogenesis of HPV infection. Further studies investigating the presence of the virus, its type, and its viral load in the examined patients are needed, in order to establish the exact role of sRAGE in HPV infection. Our findings open new perspectives and pave the way for the investigation of sRAGE in HPV infection.

Currently, there is no data available in the literature on the implication of sRAGE in the deep mechanisms that mediate the appearance and evolution of warts. These findings could help broaden the therapeutic options for HPV lesions. Some studies have shown that sRAGE could be an effective therapeutic target and might be used as a biological agent [21]. It has been suggested that increased concentrations of sRAGE may contribute to the inhibition of the inflammatory signaling pathways [47].

5. Conclusions

Our study reveals an imbalance between prooxidants and antioxidants in patients with warts. Moreover, we postulate that sRAGE may represent a potential biomarker of oxidative stress in patients with warts. sRAGE acts as a decoy for AGEs, blocking AGEs-RAGE axis and prevent the augmentation of the oxidative processes. The modulation of sRAGE could be a therapeutic alternative or at least an adjuvant treatment in near future.

Author Contributions: All authors have equally contributed to this paper. Conceptualization, C.I.M., I.N., M.T. and M.I.M.; data curation, C.C., M.I.S. and A.C.I.; formal analysis, M.I.S. and C.M.; funding acquisition, C.C.; investigation, C.D.E., C.M. and A.C.I.; methodology, C.I.M., I.N. and M.I.M.; project administration, S.R.G. and M.I.P.; resources, C.C.; software, M.T. and C.D.E.; supervision, S.R.G. and M.I.P.; validation, M.I.S., C.D.E. and C.M.; visualization, A.C.I. and S.R.G.; writing—original draft, C.I.M., I.N. and M.I.M.; writing—review and editing, M.T. and M.I.P.

Funding: This research and APC were funded by a grant of Romanian Ministry of Research and Innovation, CCCDI-UEFISCDI, [project number 61PCCDI/2018 PN-III-P1-1.2-PCCDI-2017-0341], within PNCDI-III.

Conflicts of Interest: The authors declare no conflict of interest.

References

1. Kirnbauer, R.; Androphy, E.J. Human papilloma virus infections. In *Fitzpatrick's Dermatology in General Medicine*, 8th ed.; Goldsmith, L.A., Katz, S.I., Eds.; Mc. Graw-Hill Medical: New York, NY, USA, 2012; Volume 1, pp. 2421–2433.
2. Doorbar, J.; Egawa, N.; Griffin, H.; Kranjec, C.; Murakami, I. Human papillomavirus molecular biology and disease association. *Rev. Med. Virol.* **2015**, *25* (Suppl. S1), 2–23. [CrossRef] [PubMed]
3. Harden, M.E.; Munger, K. Human papillomavirus molecular biology. *Mutat. Res. Rev. Mutat. Res.* **2017**, *772*, 3–12. [CrossRef] [PubMed]
4. Bruggink, S.C.; de Koning, M.N.; Gussekloo, J.; Egberts, P.F.; Ter Schegget, J.; Feltkamp, M.C.; Bavinck, J.N.; Quint, W.G.; Assendelft, W.J.; Eekhof, J.A. Cutaneous wart-associated HPV types: Prevalence and relation with patient characteristics. *J. Clin. Virol.* **2012**, *55*, 250–255. [CrossRef] [PubMed]
5. Cubie, H.A. Diseases associated with human papillomavirus infection. *Virology* **2013**, *445*, 21–34. [CrossRef] [PubMed]
6. Witchey, D.J.; Witchey, N.B.; Roth-Kauffman, M.M.; Kauffman, M.K. Plantar warts: Epidemiology, pathophysiology, and clinical management. *J. Am. Osteopath. Assoc.* **2018**, *118*, 92–105. [CrossRef] [PubMed]
7. Olia, J.B.H.; Ansari, M.H.K.; Yaghmaei, P.; Ayatollahi, H.; Khalkhali, H.R. Evaluation of oxidative stress marker in patients with papilloma virus infection. *Ann. TMPH* **2017**, *10*, 1518–1523.
8. Nicolae, I.; Tampa, M.; Mitran, C.; Ene, C.D.; Mitran, M.; Matei, C.; Musetescu, A.; Pituru, S.; Pop, C.S.; Georgescu, S.R. Gamma-Glutamyl Transpeptidase Alteration As A Biomarker Of Oxidative Stress in Patients with Human Papillomavirus Lesions Following Topical Treatment with Sinecatechins. *Farmacia* **2017**, *65*, 617–623.
9. Georgescu, S.R.; Mitran, C.I.; Mitran, M.I.; Caruntu, C.; Sarbu, M.I.; Matei, C.; Nicolae, I.; Tocut, S.M.; Popa, M.I.; Tampa, M. New Insights in the Pathogenesis of HPV Infection and the Associated Carcinogenic Processes: The Role of Chronic Inflammation and Oxidative Stress. *J. Immunol. Res.* **2018**, *2018*, 5315816. [CrossRef] [PubMed]
10. Cardoso, J.C.; Calonje, E. Cutaneous manifestations of human papillomaviruses: A review. *Acta Dermatovenerol. Alp. Pannonica Adriat.* **2011**, *20*, 145–154.
11. Chow, L.T.; Broker, T.R. Human papillomavirus infections: Warts or cancer? *Cold Spring Harb. Perspect. Biol.* **2013**, *5*, a012997. [CrossRef]
12. Choi, Y.J.; Park, J.S. Clinical significance of human papillomavirus genotyping. *J. Gynecol. Oncol.* **2016**, *27*, e21. [CrossRef] [PubMed]
13. Moerman-Herzog, A.; Nakagawa, M. Early defensive mechanisms against human papillomavirus infection. *Clin. Vaccine Immunol.* **2015**, *22*, 850–857. [CrossRef] [PubMed]
14. Santilli, F.; Vazzana, N.; Bucciarelli, L.G.; Davì, G. Soluble forms of RAGE in human diseases: Clinical and therapeutical implications. *Curr. Med. Chem.* **2009**, *16*, 940–952. [CrossRef] [PubMed]
15. Tang, D.; Kang, R.; Coyne, C.B.; Zeh, H.J.; Lotze, M.T. PAMPs and DAMPs: Signal 0s that spur autophagy and immunity. *Immunol. Rev.* **2012**, *249*, 158–175. [CrossRef]
16. Abeck, D.; Fölster-Holst, R. Quadrivalent human papillomavirus vaccination: A promising treatment for recalcitrant cutaneous warts in children. *Acta Derm. Venereol.* **2015**, *95*, 1017–1019. [CrossRef]

17. Iwamura, M.; Yamamoto, Y.; Kitayama, Y.; Higuchi, K.; Fujimura, T.; Hase, T.; Yamamoto, H. Epidermal expression of receptor for advanced glycation end products (RAGE) is related to inflammation and apoptosis in human skin. *Exp. Dermatol.* **2016**, *25*, 235–237. [CrossRef]
18. Papagrigoraki, A.; Maurelli, M.; Del Giglio, M.; Gisondi, P.; Girolomoni, G. Advanced Glycation End Products in the Pathogenesis of Psoriasis. *Int. J. Mol. Sci.* **2017**, *18*, 2471. [CrossRef]
19. Pranal, T.; Pereira, B.; Berthelin, P.; Roszyk, L.; Godet, T.; Chabanne, R.; Eisenmann, N.; Lautrette, A.; Belville, C.; Blondonnet, R. Clinical and Biological Predictors of Plasma Levels of Soluble RAGE in Critically Ill Patients: Secondary Analysis of a Prospective Multicenter Observational Study. *Dis. Markers* **2018**, *2018*, 7849675. [CrossRef]
20. Georgescu, S.R.; Ene, C.D.; Tampa, M.; Matei, C.; Benea, V.; Nicolae, I. Oxidative stress-related markers and alopecia areata through latex turbidimetric immunoassay method. *Mater. Plast.* **2016**, *53*, 522–526.
21. Bongarzone, S.; Savickas, V.; Luzi, F.; Gee, A.D. Targeting the receptor for advanced glycation endproducts (RAGE): A medicinal chemistry perspective. *J. Med. Chem.* **2017**, *60*, 7213–7232. [CrossRef]
22. Khan, M.I.; Su, Y.K.; Zou, J.; Yang, L.W.; Chou, R.H.; Yu, C. S100B as an antagonist to block the interaction between S100A1 and the RAGE V domain. *PLoS ONE* **2018**, *13*, e0190545. [CrossRef] [PubMed]
23. Fishman, S.L.; Sonmez, H.; Basman, C.; Singh, V.; Poretsky, L. The role of advanced glycation end-products in the development of coronary artery disease in patients with and without diabetes mellitus: A review. *Mol. Med.* **2018**, *24*, 59. [CrossRef] [PubMed]
24. Schmidt, A.M.; Yan, S.D.; Yan, S.F.; Stern, D.M. The biology of the receptor for advanced glycation end products and its ligands. *Biochim. Biophys. Acta* **2000**, *1498*, 99–111. [CrossRef]
25. van Zoelen, M.A.; Achouiti, A.; van der Poll, T. The role of receptor for advanced glycation endproducts (RAGE) in infection. *Crit. Care* **2011**, *15*, 208. [CrossRef]
26. Bierhaus, A.; Humpert, P.M.; Morcos, M.; Wendt, T.; Chavakis, T.; Arnold, B.; Stern, D.M.; Nawroth, P.P. Understanding RAGE, the receptor for advanced glycation end products. *J. Mol. Med.* **2005**, *83*, 876–886. [CrossRef]
27. Jensen, L.J.; Flyvbjerg, A.; Bjerre, M. Soluble receptor for advanced glycation end product: A biomarker for acute coronary syndrome. *BioMed Res. Int.* **2015**, *2015*, 815942. [CrossRef]
28. Meerwaldt, R.; Links, T.; Zeebregts, C.; Tio, R.; Hillebrands, J.L.; Smit, A. The clinical relevance of assessing advanced glycation endproducts accumulation in diabetes. *Cardiovasc. Diabetol.* **2008**, *7*, 29. [CrossRef]
29. Manigrasso, M.B.; Pan, J.; Rai, V.; Zhang, J.; Reverdatto, S.; Quadri, N.; DeVita, R.J.; Ramasamy, R.; Shekhtman, A.; Schmidt, A.M. Small molecule inhibition of ligand-stimulated RAGE-DIAPH1 signal transduction. *Sci. Rep.* **2016**, *6*, 22450. [CrossRef]
30. Maruthur, N.M.; Li, M.; Halushka, M.K.; Astor, B.C.; Pankow, J.S.; Boerwinkle, E.; Coresh, J.; Selvin, E.; Kao, W.H. Genetics of plasma soluble receptor for advanced glycation end-products and cardiovascular outcomes in a community-based population: Results from the Atherosclerosis Risk in Communities Study. *PLoS ONE* **2015**, *10*, e0128452. [CrossRef]
31. Vazzana, N.; Santilli, F.; Cuccurullo, C.; Davì, G. Soluble forms of RAGE in internal medicine. *Intern. Emerg. Med.* **2009**, *4*, 389–401. [CrossRef]
32. Ardans, J.A.; Eonou, A.P.; Martins, J.M.; Zhou, M.; Wahl, L.M. Oxidized low-density and high-density lipoproteins regulate the production of matrix metalloproteinase-1 and -9 by activated monocytes. *J. Leukoc. Biol.* **2002**, *71*, 1012–1018. [PubMed]
33. Yan, S.F.; Ramasamy, R.; Schmidt, A.M. Soluble RAGE: Therapy and biomarker in unraveling the RAGE axis in chronic disease and aging. *Biochem. Pharmacol.* **2010**, *79*, 1379–1386. [CrossRef] [PubMed]
34. Massaccesi, L.; Bonomelli, B.; Marazzi, M.G.; Drago, L.; Romanelli, M.M.C.; Erba, D.; Papini, N.; Barassi, A.; Goi, G.; Galliera, E. Plasmatic Soluble Receptor for Advanced Glycation End Products as a New Oxidative Stress Biomarker in Patients with Prosthetic-Joint-Associated Infections? *Dis. Markers* **2017**, *2017*, 1–7. [CrossRef] [PubMed]
35. Matsumoto, H.; Matsumoto, N.; Ogura, H.; Shimazaki, J.; Yamakawa, K.; Yamamoto, K.; Shimazu, T. The clinical significance of circulating soluble RAGE in patients with severe sepsis. *J. Trauma Acute Care Surg.* **2015**, *78*, 1086–1093. [CrossRef] [PubMed]
36. Reis, J.S.; Veloso, C.A.; Volpe, C.M.; Fernandes, J.S.; Borges, E.A.; Isoni, C.A.; Dos Anjos, P.M.; Nogueira-Machado, J.A. Soluble RAGE and malondialdehyde in type 1 diabetes patients without chronic complications during the course of the disease. *Diabete Vasc. Dis. Res.* **2012**, *9*, 309–314. [CrossRef] [PubMed]

37. Gkogkolou, P.; Böhm, M. Advanced glycation end products: Key players in skin aging? *Dermatoendocrinology* **2012**, *4*, 259–270. [CrossRef]
38. Kasperska-Zajac, A.; Damasiewicz-Bodzek, A.; Tyrpień-Golder, K.; Zamlyński, J.; Grzanka, A. Circulating soluble receptor for advanced glycation end products is decreased and inversely associated with acute phase response in chronic spontaneous urticaria. *Inflamm. Res.* **2016**, *65*, 343–346. [CrossRef]
39. Giuliano, A.R.; Siegel, E.M.; Roe, D.J.; Ferreira, S.; Baggio, M.L.; Galan, L.; Duarte-Franco, E.; Villa, L.L.; Rohan, T.E.; Marshall, J.R.; et al. Dietary intake and risk of persistent human papillomavirus (HPV) infection: The Ludwig-McGill HPV Natural History Study. *J. Infect. Dis.* **2003**, *188*, 1508–1516. [CrossRef]
40. Briganti, S.; Picardo, M. Antioxidant activity, lipid peroxidation and skin diseases. What's new. *J. Eur. Acad. Dermatol. Venereol.* **2003**, *17*, 663–669. [CrossRef]
41. Erturan, I.; Kumbul Doğuç, D.; Korkmaz, S.; Büyükbayram, H.İ.; Yıldırım, M.; Kocabey Uzun, S. Evaluation of oxidative stress in patients with recalcitrant warts. *J. Eur. Acad. Dermatol. Venereol.* **2019**, *33*, jdv.15746. [CrossRef]
42. Tampa, M.; Nicolae, I.L.; Ene, C.D.; Sarbu, I.; Matei, C.L.; Georgescu, S.R. Vitamin C and thiobarbituric acid reactive substances (TBARS) in psoriasis vulgaris related to psoriasis area severity index (PASI). *Rev. Chim.* **2017**, *68*, 43–47.
43. Hudson, B.I.; Moon, Y.P.; Kalea, A.Z.; Khatri, M.; Marquez, C.; Schmidt, A.M.; Paik, M.C.; Yoshita, M.; Sacco, R.L.; DeCarli, C.; et al. Association of serum soluble receptor for advanced glycation end-products with subclinical cerebrovascular disease: The Northern Manhattan Study (NOMAS). *Atherosclerosis* **2011**, *216*, 192–198. [CrossRef] [PubMed]
44. Mitran, M.I.; Mitran, C.I.; Sarbu, M.I.; Matei, C.; Nicolae, I.; Caruntu, A.; Tocut, S.M.; Popa, M.I.; Caruntu, C.; Georgescu, S.R. Mediators of Inflammation–A Potential Source of Biomarkers in Oral Squamous Cell Carcinoma. *J. Immunol. Res.* **2018**, *2018*, 1061780.
45. McNair, E.D.; Wells, C.R.; Mabood Qureshi, A.; Basran, R.; Pearce, C.; Orvold, J.; Devilliers, J.; Prasad, K. Modulation of high sensitivity C-reactive protein by soluble receptor for advanced glycation end products. *Mol. Cell. Biochem.* **2010**, *341*, 135–138. [CrossRef] [PubMed]
46. Sasmaz, S.; Arican, O.; Kurutas, E.B. Oxidative stress in patients with nongenital warts. *Mediat. Inflamm.* **2005**, *2005*, 233–236. [CrossRef] [PubMed]
47. Yonchuk, J.G.; Silverman, E.K.; Bowler, R.P.; Agustí, A.; Lomas, D.A.; Miller, B.E.; Tal-Singer, R.; Mayer, R.J. Circulating soluble receptor for advanced glycation end products (sRAGE) as a biomarker of emphysema and the RAGE axis in the lung. *Am. J. Respir. Crit. Care Med.* **2015**, *192*, 785–792. [CrossRef]

medicina

MDPI

Article

Hepatitis B Virus Genotypes in the Kingdom of Bahrain: Prevalence, Gender Distribution and Impact on Hepatic Biomarkers

Essam M. Janahi [1,*], Zahra Ilyas [1], Sara Al-Othman [2], Abdulla Darwish [3], Sanad J. Sanad [4], Budoor Almusaifer [3], Mariam Al-Mannai [5], Jamal Golbahar [6] and Simone Perna [1,*]

1 Department of Biology, College of Science, University of Bahrain, Shakir P.O. Box 32038, Bahrain; zahra.muhammadilyas@gmail.com

2 Molecular Diagnostic Al-Jawhara Centre for Molecular Medicine and Inherited Disorders, AGU, Manama 329, Bahrain; sarash@agu.edu.bh

3 Department of Pathology, Bahrain Defense Force Hospital, West Riffa P.O. Box 28743, Bahrain; abdulla.darwish660@gmail.com (A.D.); b.mm89@hotmail.com (B.A.)

4 Department of Internal Medicine, Bahrain Defense Hospital, West Riffa P.O. Box 28743, Bahrain; Sanad.jassim@outlook.com

5 Department of Mathematics, College of Science, University of Bahrain, Shakir P.O. Box 32038, Bahrain; malmannai@uob.edu.bh

6 Department of Clinical Biochemistry, Northern Devon NHS Trust, North Devon District Hospital, Barnstaple EX31 4JB, UK; jgolbahar@nhs.net

* Correspondence: essam22@gmail.com (E.M.J.); simoneperna@hotmail.it (S.P.); Tel.: +973-1743-7425 (E.M.J.); +973-39-37-99-46 (S.P.); Fax: +973-1744-9662 (E.M.J.)

Received: 8 July 2019; Accepted: 16 September 2019; Published: 23 September 2019

Abstract: *Background*: Approximately 400 million people are infected with Hepatitis B virus (HBV) around the world, which makes it one of the world's major infectious diseases. The prevalence of HBV genotypes and predictive factors for risk are poorly known in the Kingdom of Bahrain. *Objectives*: The aim of the present study was to investigate the prevalence of HBV genotypes, its correlation with demographic factor sand impacts on hepatic biomarkers. *Materials and Methods*: Venous blood samples were collected from 82 HBV positive patients (48 males, 34 females). The extraction of HBV DNA, PCR amplification, and genotyping were done to classify different genotypes (A, A/D, B, B/D, C, D, D/E, E). HBV genotypes association with gender, nationality, mode of transmission, and liver cirrhosis complication was determined by descriptive statistic and univariate analysis of variance (ANOVA). For liver function test, unpaired t-test and ANOVA were performed. *Results:* The predominant genotype among patients under study was genotype D (61%), followed by genotype A (10%), and lowest frequency was found for undetermined genotype (1%). In general, there was no significant association between the different genotypes and some demographical factors, serological investigations, and liver function test. The prevalence of HBV genotypes was higher in male patients as compared to female patients and higher in non-Bahraini than in Bahraini. Patients with the dominant genotype D showed higher than the normal maximum range for alanine aminotransferase (ALT) (mean = 45.89) and Gamma-glutamyl transferase (GGT) (mean = 63.36). *Conclusions*: The most common HBV genotype in Bahrain was genotype D, followed by genotype A. Further studies involving the sources of transmission and impact of hepatic biomarker in Bahrain are required to enhance the control measures of HBV infections.

Keywords: prevalence; hepatitis B virus; genotype; bahrain

1. Introduction

Hepatitis B Virus (HBV) is chronically carried by around 400 million people worldwide and about one million die annually as result of developing liver cirrhosis and hepatocellular carcinoma [1–3]. The infection is mainly present in Middle East, South-East Asia, sub-Saharan Africa, Central and South-America, and Eastern-Europe with prevalence >8% of population [4]. A migratory flow that had occurred in last twenty years from these countries to the industrialized countries resulted in an increase in HBV prevalence the industrialized countries [1,5]. Between 5 and 10% of infected individuals become chronic carriers in their adulthood, while 85 to 95% in their infancy [6].

Hepatitis B virus is transmitted through blood and body fluids, hence certain types of behaviors increase the risk of infection, such as sharing personal items (toothbrushes, razors, etc.), use of contaminant needles for intravenous drugs or ear pricing and tattooing, and practicing unsafe sex. Hemodialysis and hemophiliacs patients as well as Healthcare and emergency service workers are also at higher risk [7].

HBV genome has a high rate of mutation when compared to other DNA viruses due to the high spontaneous error rate of the viral reverse transcriptase and lack of proofreading mechanism. It is estimated approximately 1.4–3.2 $\times 10^{-5}$ per genome. Accordingly, HBV can be classified into eight genotypes A-H that accounts for 8% or more in the complete nucleotide sequence on inter-sequence divergence [8,9]. Studies on HBV genotypes show a distinct geographical distribution around the world [10]. In general, genotype A is pandemic, but most prevalent in North West Europe, North America, Central Africa [11], and India [8,12]. Genotypes B and C are prevalent in Asia [1,13], especially in the populations of Eastern Asia and the Far East [3]. Genotype D is distributed worldwide with the highest prevalence in the Mediterranean region [3,9,14]. Genotype E and F are predominant in West Africa and in the Amerindian population, respectively [1,9,13]. Recently, genotype G was identified in the USA and France [1]. Genotype H was also recently found in Central America [15]. A remarkable difference in the clinical and virologic characteristics between the patients with different genotypes has been reported [2].

HBV genotypes are reported to be responsible for the differences in the natural history of chronic infection and they play a significant role in clinical manifestation of infection and response to antiviral therapy [16]. Therapeutically, patients that are infected with genotypes A, B, D, and F show frequent spontaneous HBeAg seroconversion when compared to genotype C. Whereas, patients that were infected with genotype E have higher frequency of HBeAg positivity and higher viral loads as compared to patients that were infected with genotype D [17].

Epidemiological data regarding HBV in any country would provide significant information to program managers and health planers to control and manage the infection with reference to its etiological spectrum. In the present study, we aim to determine the prevalence of the various HBV genotypes in the Kingdom of Bahrain. This study also aims to determine various sociodemographic factors and hepatic biomarker associated with the prevalence and the possible risk factors for HBV transmission in Bahrain.

2. Method

2.1. Setting

Bahrain is a small archipelago country (33 islands) that is situated near the western shores of the Arabian Gulf with a total area of 765.3 km^2. It has a total population of 1,234,571, out of which 666,172 are non-Bahraini and it is one of the most densely populated countries in the world (1461/km^2) [18].

2.2. Study Design

In this cross-sectional study, patients with established chronic hepatitis B infection (positive for HBsAg antigen, HBcAg antibody) referred to Bahrain Defense Force Hospital (second largest hospital in Bahrain) were investigated for HBV genotypes. The major inclusion criterion was testing positive for HBsAg for over six months (chronic infection), with levels of ALT around the normal range. All patients were negative for antibodies against hepatitis C and human immunodeficiency virus.

2.3. Sample Collection, HBV DNA Extraction and Genotyping

Five ml of venous blood were collected from patients and sera were separated and stored at −80 °C prior to HBV genotyping. HBV DNA extraction, PCR amplification of DNA, and genotyping were carried out according to the instruction while using a commercially available kit (SMITEST, MBL Co. Nogoya, Japan) based on hybridization with type-specific probes immobilized on a solid-phase support. The quality and quantity of extracted DNA was determined with a Nano drop spectrophotometer (Thermo Scientific, Wilmington, DE, USA) after DNA extraction. Serological investigation for HBsAg and HBeAg were carried out while using commercial enzyme-linked immunosorbent assay (ELISA) kits (ARCHITECT ANALYSER i2000, Abbott, Santa Clara, CA, USA). Liver function tests; Total and Direct Bilirubin, Alanine Transaminase (ALT), Alkaline Phosphatase (ALP), Aspartate Transaminase (AST), Gama Glutamyl Transferase (γGT) and Lactate Dehydrogenase (LDH) were analyzed in serum samples while using routine biochemistry analyzer (COBAS c 501, Roche/ Mannheim, Germany).

2.4. Statistical Analysis

Statistical analyses were performed while using IBM SPSS Statistics 23 software. For baseline variables, summary statistics employed frequencies data, mean, and standard deviation (SD) for continuous variables. Continuous variables were compared using unpaired t-tests and ANOVA as appropriate. Descriptive Statistics were calculated to determine the prevalence of genotype with respect to data of demographic factors, serology, and other investigations. Univariate analysis of Variance (ANOVA) was applied to determine any significance differences for the genotype and liver function tests.

2.5. Ethical Approval

The local ethics and research committees of Bahrain Defense Force Hospital and University of Bahrain approved this study (approval date 7 September 2017, Project code: 2017/12). It conformed to the provisions of the Declaration of Helsinki in 1964 (and revised in Fortaleza, Brazil, October 2013). All of the patients signed the informed consent form before participation.

3. Results

3.1. Demographic Characteristics of Patients

Eighty-two HBV positive patients (48 males, 34 females), were screened for the different genotypes A, B, C, D, E and mixed genotype infections A/D, B/D, D/E. The patients in the study were either Bahraini nationals or from other nationalities. The frequency of Bahraini was found to be 53.7% and that of Non-Bahraini was 46.3%. The highest prevalence of HBV infection was shown for the age group 21–30. The lowest prevalence was for the group <21. There was no significance difference between genotype and nationality, gender and age-group ($p > 0.05$), as shown in Table 1.

Table 1. Sociodemographic factors associated with the prevalence of hepatitis B virus infections examined patients (N = 82).

Variables	No. of Isolation [1]	*p*-Value
Gender		0.447
Male	58.5 (48)	
Female	41.5 (34)	
Nationality		0.44
Bahraini	53.7 (44)	
Non-Bahraini	46.3 (38)	
Age-group		0.409
<21	4.9 (4)	
21–30	28 (23)	
31–40	25.6 (21)	
41–50	13.4(11)	
51–60	15.9(13)	
>61	12.2(10)	

[1] Data presented as %(No.).

3.2. Distribution of HBV Genotypes in the Study Population

Figure 1 illustrates the frequency of HBV genotypes A, A/D, B, B/D, C, D, D/E, and E. The prevalence of genotype A was found to be 10%, genotype A/B was 7%, genotype B was 4%, genotype B/D was 2%, genotype C was 5%, genotype D/E was 4%, genotype E was 1%, and undetermined genotypes was 6%. Among the referred genotypes, genotype D showed the highest occurrence (61%), which indicated that genotype D is the most prevalent HBV genotype in the Kingdom of Bahrain.

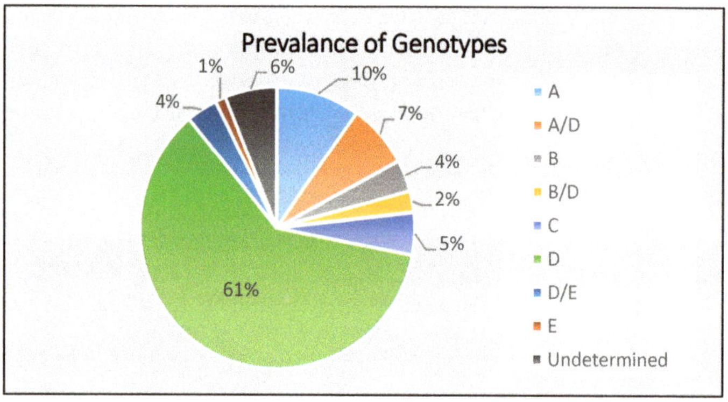

Figure 1. Prevalence of HBV genotypes among 82 patients under study in the Kingdom of Bahrain.

3.3. Genotype and Sociodemographic Data

Table 2 states the distribution of genotypes with respect to gender, nationality, and age groups. The prevalence of HBV infection for each genotype differs for gender, but there is no significance difference in terms of genotype prevalence and genders ($p = 0.447$; $p > 0.05$). Overall, the genotype A (62.5%), A/D (66.7%), B (66.7%), C (100%), and D/E (100%) are more related to males, whereas genotype E (100%) and Undetermined genotype (60%) are more related to females. Genotype A/D (66.7%), D (64.0%), and Undetermined genotypes (80%) are more related to Bahraini nationality; Genotype A (87.5%), B (6.7%), C (75%), D/E (100%), and E (100%) are more related to other nationalities. Genotype B/D (50%) is equally distributed among and Bahrainis and non-Bahrainis. Individuals of different age groups were enrolled in the study, there was no significance differences in terms of genotype prevalence and age ($p = 0.409$; $p > 0.05$).

3.4. HBV Genotype Relationship with Mode of Transmission and Liver Cirrhosis Complications

Table 3 shows the prevalence of HBV genotypes in relationship to the mode of transmission and liver cirrhosis complications. There are no significant differences ($p > 0.05$) in genotype frequency in relation to the mode of transmission ($p = 0.086$) and liver cirrhosis complications ($p = 0.857$). Genotype A (37.5%), A/D (66.7%), D (66%), D/E (100%), and undetermined genotype (80%) are more related to the unknown factor of infection transmission. Genotype B (66.7%) and C (75.5%) are more related to Blood transfusion while genotype E (100%) is more related to vertical transmission from mother to child. Genotype D (2%) is more related to hemodialysis, while genotype A (12.5%) is more related to tattoo/body piercing. In general, there was low or no relationship between the prevalence of HBV genotypes and liver cirrhosis complications, for example, genotype A (50%), genotype A/D (66.7%), genotype B (100%), genotype C (100%), genotype D (78%), genotype D/E (100%), and undetermined (80%), except for mixed genotypes B/D, 50% of the patients were associated with ascites.

Table 2. Prevalence of Hepatitis B Virus (HBV) Genotypes in Patients of Different Gender, Age and Nationality (N = 82).

	Gender		Nationality		Age-Group					
Genotype	**Male (48)**	**Female (34)**	**Bahraini (44)**	**Non-Bahraini (38)**	**<20 (4)**	**21–30 (23)**	**31–40 (21)**	**41–50 (11)**	**51–60 (13)**	**>61 (10)**
A	62.5%	37.5%	12.5%	87.5%	0.0%	25.0%	25.0%	25.0%	12.5%	12.5%
A/D	66.7%	33.3%	66.7%	33.3%	0.0%	83.3%	16.7%	0.0%	0.0%	0.0%
B	66.7%	33.3%	33.3%	66.7%	0.0%	0.0%	33.3%	0.0%	33.3%	33.3%
B/D	50.0%	50.0%	50.0%	50.0%	0.0%	0.0%	100.0%	0.0%	0.0%	0.0%
C	100.0%	0.0%	25.0%	75.0%	0.0%	25.0%	50.0%	25.0%	0.0%	0.0%
D	54.0%	46.0%	64.0%	36.0%	8.0%	22.0%	20.0%	14.0%	22.0%	14.0%
D/E	100.0%	0.0%	0.0%	100.0%	0.0%	100.0%	0.0%	0.0%	0.0%	0.0%
E	0.0%	100.0%	0.0%	100.0%	0.0%	100.0%	0.0%	0.0%	0.0%	0.0%
Undetermined	40.0%	60.0%	80.0%	20.0%	0.0%	0.0%	60.0%	20.0%	0.0%	20.0%

Table 3. Frequency of HBV Genotypes in Correlation with Mode of Transmission and Liver Cirrhosis Complications.

	Mode of Transmission					Liver Cirrhosis				
Genotype	**Unknown (49)**	**Blood/Blood Products (16)**	**Sexual (6)**	**Maternal/Vertical (6)**	**Organ Transplant (3)**	**None (63)**	**Ascites (13)**	**Portal HTn (2)**	**HCC (2)**	**Hepatic Encephalopathy (2)**
A	37.50%	12.50%	25.00%	12.50%	0.00%	50.00%	37.50%	12.50%	0.00%	0.00%
A/D	66.70%	16.70%	0.00%	0.00%	16.70%	66.70%	0.00%	0.00%	16.70%	16.70%
B	0.00%	66.70%	0.00%	0.00%	33.30%	100.00%	0.00%	0.00%	0.00%	0.00%
B/D	50.00%	0.00%	50.00%	0.00%	0.00%	50.00%	50.00%	0.00%	0.00%	0.00%
C	25.00%	75.00%	0.00%	0.00%	0.00%	100.00%	0.00%	0.00%	0.00%	0.00%
D	66.00%	16.00%	6.00%	8.00%	2.00%	78.00%	16.00%	2.00%	2.00%	2.00%
D/E	100.00%	0.00%	0.00%	0.00%	0.00%	100.00%	0.00%	0.00%	0.00%	0.00%
E	0.00%	0.00%	0.00%	100.00%	0.00%	100.00%	0.00%	0.00%	0.00%	0.00%
Undetermined	80.00%	20.00%	0.00%	0.00%	0.00%	80.00%	20.00%	0.00%	0.00%	0.00%

3.5. HBV Genotype and Liver Function Test

For the determination of HBV clinical course, investigating the hepatic biomarkers plays an important role. As increase or decrease in their levels can indicate hepatic disfunction. Bilirubin, Direct Bilirubin (Dbilirubin), Alanine transaminase (ALT), Aspartate aminotransferase (AST), and Gamma-Glutamyl Transferase (GGT) were measured and associated with the different genotypes. Table 4 summaries the mean and SD values in relation to the different genotypes. The maximum and minimum range for these liver function enzymes were stated as: Bilirubin (max. 17, min. 0 umol/L), Dbilirubin (max. 3.4, min. 0 umol/L), AST (max. 37, min. 0 IU/L), ALT (max. 41, min. 0 IU/L), and GGT (max. 49, min. 11 IU/L). Table 4 shows that for Bilirubin value A/D mixed genotype was higher than the max range; for D bilirubin, no genotypes were above or below the normal range, while for AST, ALT, and GGT, the genotypes A, A/D, B, and B/D were all above the normal range.

Table 4. Mean and Standard Deviation of Liver Function Tests, Univariate Analysis with HBV Genotype.

Genotypes	Bilirubin (umol/L)	Dbilirubin (umol/L)	AST (IU/L)	ALT (IU/L)	GGT (IU/L)
A	14.39 (±3.65)	6.94 (±2.81)	44.04 * (±3.78)	49.54 * (±8.77)	65.75 * (±23.22)
A/D	25.10 * (±8.48)	12.78 (±4.79)	77.43 * (±3.68)	94.23 * (±8.89)	65.33 * (±28.07)
B	16.63 (±12.35)	8.97 (±6.77)	35.40 (±14.61)	63.93 * (±38.93)	60.00 * (±39.68)
B/D	16.35 (±11.05)	10.55 (±8.35)	69.40 * (±0.00)	86.90 * (±69.80)	76.00 * (±67.00)
C	6.68 (±2.18)	1.93 (±0.39)	20.45 (±3.15)	21.53 (±5.97)	41.25 (±15.26)
D	13.26 (±1.51)	6.09 (±0.62)	31.76 (±3.05)	45.89 * (±6.60)	63.36 * (±2.68)
D/E	7.70 (±2.99)	3.30 (±1.14)	24.93 (±3.58)	33.53 (±6.63)	25.33 (± 7.88)
E	3.20 (±0.00)	1.50 (±0.00)	37.00 * (±0.00)	44.50 * (±0.00)	15.00 (±0.00)
Undetermined	7.14 (±1.41)	2.50 (±0.25)	18.80 (±2.69)	21.32 (±4.45)	18.00 (±4.06)

* Refers to the measured levels of the liver functions enzymes above their min. and max. ranges.

4. Discussion

HBV infection is an important global problem that places a continuously increasing burden on developing countries. As the HBV genotype can be classified into different genotypes, the classification has to be cost-effective and clinically relevant [19]. Research on the relationship between HBV genotypes, their pathogenicity in chronic liver disease, including hepatocellular carcinoma, and their therapy are of great interest, as this allows for understanding the spread and risk of HBV infection around the world [10]. On the other hand, HBV infection is a major health problem in the Middle East. The majority of the countries in the region have an intermediate or high endemicity of HBV infection [20]. Despite the low prevalence of HBV in Bahrain, it is important to investigate the frequency of HBV genotypes and its association with various sociodemographic factors, hepatic biomarkers, and mode of transmission, which is essential for fine tuning the control of the disease.

According to a study by Janahi (2014), completed on 877,892 individuals, Bahrain has low HBV endemicity for the period (2000–2010). The prevalence of hepatitis B virus infection in Bahrain was found to be 0.58% [21]. This study reports for the first time in Bahrain, the correlation of HBV genotypes frequency with the demographic characteristics and hepatic biomarker. The results showed that there were no significant differences of genotype frequency in relation to the demographic characteristics as well as hepatic biomarkers. Out of the 82 screened patients in this study, 58.5% were male, while the remaining 41.5% were females. There was a significant increased risk of HBV infection in male as compared to females (Table 1). 53.7% of HBV positive patients had Bahraini nationality, while the remaining 46.3% belonged to other eleven nationalities, such as Pakistan, Sudan, Egypt, Yamen, Syria, Kuwait, Bangladesh, India, Ethiopia, Indonesia, and Philippines, which are known to be highly endemic for HBV. Relationship between genotype and age-group indicates that HBV prevails 4.9% in <21 years, 28% in 21–30 years, 25.6% in 31–40 years, 13.4% in 41–50 years, 15.9% in 51–60 years, and 12.2% in >61 years. age groups.

The frequency of mode of transmission was highly unknown (59.8%), followed by blood/blood products (19.5%), sexual contact (7.3%), vertical transmission (7.3%), and finally organ transplant (3.7%). HBV and HCV have common modes of transmission; therefore, their coinfection is quite frequent. This particularly occurs in areas where the two viruses are endemic and among subjects with high risk of parental infection [22]. According to a study that was conducted in Bahrain, dental procedures and surgical operations account for 37.2% and 35.6%, respectively, of the HBV transmission routes. Followed by the blood transfusion (24.6%), the sexual contact and intervenors drug abuse were the least possible routes of transmission [21]. There was some significant difference in the HBV genotype prevalence with respect to some investigated variables. For example, the frequency of HBV genotype is more related to males and the risk of HBV infection increased with older age.

The dominant genotype in our study was genotype D with 61% frequency, which is similar to some countries in the Middle East, like Saudi Arabia (81%) [23], UAE (79.5%) [24], Iran, and Jordan (≈100%) [25,26]. The dominance of this genotype might be attributed to different factors, such as the presence of high number of workers from countries that are known to have dominant D genotype, such as India, Pakistan, Yemen, Syria, and Bangladesh. These infected workers are a principal source for the transmission of hepatitis B. As most of them belong to highly endemic countries with low educational and socio-economical backgrounds, they positively contribute to the transmission of the disease. Living in small houses and having unhygienic behaviors (such as sharing same razors and toothbrushes) put such workers at high risk of contracting HBV. A poor hygiene system in hospitals of such countries is known as a high-risk factor for HBV transmission, as the same syringe is used for vaccination of different people [27].

The quasi-species nature of HBV infection indicates that the variation and evolution of Hepatitis B virus has been influenced by the recombination between genotypes. Hence, a high prevalence of more than one dominant genotype in a certain region is common [16,28]. It is documented that mixed infection with different HBV genotypes is not uncommon and it is of great virological and clinical interest. For example, a study done by Chen et al. (2004) showed that the prevalence of mixed HBV genotype infection was 16.3% for HBsAg positive and 34.4% in occult HBV-infected intravenous drug users [29].

HBV is non-cytopathic virus, which highlights the complex and important interaction between the virus and host in causing HBV-related liver disease. Bilirubin, Direct Bilirubin, ALT, and AST are the most common liver enzymes that are measured to investigate the condition of liver due to HBV or HCV infection [30]. Elevated ALT levels, elevated AST level, elevated serum bilirubin, and decreased serum albumin might be indicative of advanced liver disease and even cirrhosis [31]. In our study, there was no significant association between HBV prevalence and liver function test. However, each genotype showed variation depending on the mean and standard deviation of the liver function test associated with that genotype. The most dominant genotype in the present study, genotype D showed high levels of ALT and GGT above the normal range. This might be indicative of acute hepatitis. Genotype A and mixed genotypes B/D showed higher than the normal maximum level for ALT, AST, and GGT; mixed genotypes A/D showed higher than the normal maximum level for Bilirubin, ALT, AST, and GGT; genotype B showed higher than the normal maximum level for ALT and GGT; genotype D showed higher than the normal maximum level for ALT and GGT; and, genotype E showed higher than the normal maximum level for AST and ALT. Genotype C and undetermined genotypes showed normal liver function enzymes levels. It is also reported that persistently elevated liver enzymes levels in an asymptomatic hepatitis B patient is associated with high infectivity [32].

This study, as any study, has some limitations. Firstly, 82 individuals only were screened, which is a relatively small sample and it may not represent an accurate picture of HBV prevalence at the population level. Secondly, no cases from other governmental and private health facilities were included in our study which may contribute to lower prevalence. However, according to the latest data that were obtained from the Public Health Directorate, Ministry of Health, the number of HBV positive patients at population level was 527, so our sample 82 represents approximately 16% of the total HBV patients in Bahrain. Thirdly, some of the obtained data from patients were based on patient self-reporting of risk factors, which is subject to social desirability bias.

Finally, this study showed that the overall HBV prevalence among males' patients to be 58.5%, while it was 41.5% among females. The dominant HBV genotype in Bahrain was genotype D (61%), which was associated with higher than the normal maximum level of ALT and GGT.

5. Conclusions

This study highlighted the importance of hepatic biomarker association with genotypes, which can be used as a base for further studies to investigate such an association. The advantage of this study was to provide a baseline study to draw a good estimate of HBV genotype distribution in Bahrain.

Author Contributions: Conceptualization, E.M.J.; methodology, S.A.-O., A.D., E.M.J., J.G., S.J.S., B.A., Z.I. and S.P.; data curation, E.M.J., M.A.-M., Z.I., and S.P.; writing—original draft preparation, E.M.J. and J.G.; writing—review and editing, E.M.J., Z.I., S.P.

Funding: This research was funded by University of Bahrain, Deanship of Scientific Research, grant number [4/2017].

Acknowledgments: The authors wish to thank all participants in this study and also to thank BDF hospital for collecting clinical samples. The authors would like also to thank Fatema Abdulwaheed Yaqub and Rukaya Abdulghafoor Jalal for their help in HBV genotyping and data entry. Finally, it is our pleasure to acknowledge with gratitude the financial support of University of Bahrain, Deanship of Scientific Research.

Conflicts of Interest: The authors declare no conflict of interest.

References

1. Kao, J.; Chen, P.; Lai, M.; Chen, D. Genotypes and Clinical Phenotypes of Hepatitis B Virus in Patients with Chronic Hepatitis B Virus Infection. *J. Clin. Microbiol.* **2002**, *40*, 1207–1209. [CrossRef] [PubMed]
2. Chan, H.; Wong, M.; Hui, A.; Hung, L.; Chan, F.; Sung, J. Hepatitis B Virus Genotype C Takes a More Aggressive Disease Course Than Hepatitis B Virus Genotype B in Hepatitis B e Antigen-Positive Patients. *J. Clin. Microbiol.* **2003**, *41*, 1277–1279. [CrossRef] [PubMed]
3. Ogawa, M. Clinical features and viral sequences of various genotypes of hepatitis B virus compared among patients with acute hepatitis B. *Hepatol. Res.* **2002**, *23*, 167–177. [CrossRef]
4. Lavanchy, D. Hepatitis B virus epidemiology, disease burden, treatment, and current and emerging prevention and control measures. *J. Viral Hepat.* **2004**, *11*, 97–107. [CrossRef] [PubMed]
5. Nicoletta, P.; Daniel, L. *Hepatitis B.*; World Health Organization: Geneva, Switzerland, 2002.
6. Zhang, X.; Zoulim, F.; Habersetzer, F.; Xiong, S.; Trépo, C. Analysis of hepatitis B virus genotypes and pre-core region variability during interferon treatment of HBe antigen negative chronic hepatitis B. *J. Med Virol.* **1996**, *48*, 8–16. [CrossRef]
7. André, F. Hepatitis B epidemiology in Asia, the Middle East and Africa. *Vaccine* **2000**, *18*, S20–S22. [CrossRef]
8. Jazayeri, M.; Basuni, A.; Sran, N.; Gish, R.; Cooksley, G.; Locarnini, S.; Carman, W. HBV core sequence: Definition of genotype-specific variability and correlation with geographical origin. *J. Viral Hepat.* **2004**, *11*, 488–501. [CrossRef]
9. Stuyver, L.; Rossau, R.; Zoulim, F.; Fried, M.; De Gendt, S.; Schinazi, R.; Van Geyt, C. A new genotype of hepatitis B virus: Complete genome and phylogenetic relatedness. *J. Gen. Virol.* **2000**, *81*, 67–74. [CrossRef]
10. Huy, T.; Abe, K. Molecular epidemiology of hepatitis B and C virus infections in Asia. *Pediatr. Int.* **2004**, *46*, 223–230. [CrossRef]
11. Van Geyt, C.; De Gendt, S.; Rombout, A.; Wyseur, A.; Maertens, G.; Bartholomeusz, A.; Schinazi, R.F.; Locarnini, S.A. Significance of mutations in the hepatitis B virus polymerase selected by nucleoside analogues and implicationfor controlling chronic disease. *Viral Hepat. Rev.* **1998**, *4*, 167–187.
12. Ding, X.; Mizokami, M.; Yao, G.; Xu, B.; Orito, E.; Ueda, R.; Nakanishi, M. Hepatitis B Virus Genotype Distribution among Chronic Hepatitis B Virus Carriers in Shanghai, China. *Intervirology* **2001**, *44*, 43–47. [CrossRef] [PubMed]

13. Sugauchi, F.; Chutaputti, A.; Orito, E.; Kato, H.; Suzuki, S.; Ueda, R.; Mizokami, M. Hepatitis B virus genotypes and clinical manifestation among hepatitis B carriers in Thailand. *J. Gastroenterol. Hepatol.* **2002**, *17*, 671–676. [CrossRef] [PubMed]
14. Magnius, L.; Norder, H. Subtypes, Genotypes and Molecular Epidemiology of the Hepatitis B Virus as Reflected by Sequence Variability of the S-Gene. *Intervirology* **1995**, *38*, 24–34. [CrossRef] [PubMed]
15. Arauz-Ruiz, P.; Norder, H.; Robertson, B.H.; Magnius, L.O. Genotype H: A new Amerindian genotype of hepatitis B virus revealed in Central America. *J. Gen. Virol.* **2002**, *83*, 2059–2073. [CrossRef] [PubMed]
16. Liaw, Y.; Brunetto, M.; Hadziyannis, S. The natural history of chronic HBV infection and geographical differences. *Antivir. Ther.* **2010**, *15*, 25–33. [CrossRef] [PubMed]
17. Kramvis, A. Genotypes and Genetic Variability of Hepatitis B Virus. *Intervirology* **2014**, *57*, 141–150. [CrossRef] [PubMed]
18. Ministry of Cabinet Affairs, Kingdom of Bahrain. *Basic Results Population, Housing, Buildings and Establishment Census*; Ministry of Cabinet Affairs, Kingdom of Bahrain: Manama, Bahrain, 2010.
19. Miyakawa, Y.; Mizokami, M. Classifying Hepatitis B Virus Genotypes. *Intervirology* **2003**, *46*, 329–338. [CrossRef] [PubMed]
20. Qirbi, N.; Hall, A.J. Epidemiology of hepatitis B virus infection in the Middle East: A Review. *La Revue de Sante de la Mediterranee Orientale* **2001**, *7*, 1034–1045.
21. Janahi, E. Prevalence and Risk Factors of Hepatitis B Virus Infection in Bahrain, 2000 through 2010. *PLoS ONE* **2014**, *9*, e87599. [CrossRef]
22. Hui, C.; Lau, E.; Monto, A.; Kim, M.; Luk, J.; Poon, R.; Wright, T.L. Natural History of Patients with Recurrent Chronic Hepatitis C Virus and Occult Hepatitis B Co-Infection after Liver Transplantation. *Am. J. Transplant.* **2006**, *6*, 1600–1608. [CrossRef]
23. Al Ashgar, H.; Peedikayil, M.; Imambaccus, H.; Althawadi, S. Prevalence of hepatitis B virus genotype in Saudi Arabia: A preliminary report. *Indian J. Gastroenterol.* **2008**, *2008*.
24. Alfaresi, M.; Elkoush, A.; Alshehhi, H.; Alzaabi, A.; Islam, A. Hepatitis B virus genotypes and precore and core mutants in UAE patients. *Virol. J.* **2010**, *7*. [CrossRef] [PubMed]
25. Alavian, S.M.; Fallahian, F.; Lankarani, K.B. The changing epidemiology of viral hepatitis B in Iran. *J. Gastrointest. Liver Dis.* **2007**, *16*, 403–406.
26. Ghazzawi, I.; Hamoudi, M.; Hamoudi, W. Hepatitis B Genotypic and Serologic Characteristics in Jordan. *J. R. Med. Serv.* **2016**, *23*, 17–22. [CrossRef]
27. Fung, S.K.; Wong, F.S.; Wong, D.K.; Hussain, M.T.; Lok, A.S. Hepatitis B virus genotypes, precore and core promoter variants among predominantly Asian patients with chronic HBV infection in a Canadian center. *Liver Int.* **2006**, *26*, 796–804. [CrossRef] [PubMed]
28. McMahon, B. The influence of hepatitis B virus genotype and subgenotype on the natural history of chronic hepatitis B. *Hepatol. Int.* **2008**, *3*, 334–342. [CrossRef]
29. Chen, C.; Hung, C.; Lee, C.; Hu, T.; Wang, J.H.; Wang, J.C.; Changchien, C.S. Pre-S Deletion and Complex Mutations of Hepatitis B Virus Related to Advanced Liver Disease in HBeAg-Negative Patients. *Gastroenterology* **2007**, *133*, 1466–1474. [CrossRef] [PubMed]
30. Hadziyannis, S.J.; Papatheodoridis, G.V. Hepatitis B e Antigen-Negative Chronic Hepatitis B: Natural History and Treatment. *Semin. Liver Dis.* **2006**, *26*, 130–141. [CrossRef]
31. Limdi, J.K.; Hyde, G.M. Evaluation of abnormal liver function tests. *Postgrad. Med. J.* **2003**, *79*, 307–312. [CrossRef]
32. Giboney, P.T. Mildly elevated liver transaminase levels in the asymptomatic patient. *Am. Fam. Phys.* **2005**, *71*, 1105–1110.

medicina

MDPI

Article

Antiviral Activity of Exopolysaccharides Produced by Lactic Acid Bacteria of the Genera *Pediococcus*, *Leuconostoc* and *Lactobacillus* against Human Adenovirus Type 5

Liubov Biliavska *, Yulia Pankivska, Olga Povnitsa and Svitlana Zagorodnya

Zabolotny Institute of Microbiology and Virology, National Academy of Sciences of Ukraine, 03143 Kyiv, Ukraine

* Correspondence: bilyavskal@ukr.net; Tel.: +38-096-301-5098

Received: 22 June 2019; Accepted: 20 August 2019; Published: 22 August 2019

Abstract: *Background and objectives*: The use of antagonistic probiotic microorganisms and their byproducts represents a promising approach for the treatment of viral diseases. In the current work, the effect of exopolysaccharides (EPSs) produced by lactic acid bacteria from different genera on the structural and functional characteristics of cells and the development of adenoviral infection in vitro was studied. *Materials and Methods:* Cytotoxicity of six EPSs of lactic acid bacteria of the genera *Lactobacillus*, *Leuconostoc* and *Pediococcus* was determined by MTT (3-(4,5-dimethylthiazol-2-yl)-2,5-diphenyl tetrazolium bromide) assay. The influence of the EPSs on the infectivity of human adenovirus type 5 (HAdV-5) and on the cell cycle under a condition of adenovirus infection was studied using plaque reduction assay and flow cytometric analysis, respectively. *Results*: It was shown that exopolysaccharides were non-toxic to Madin-Darby bovine kidney cells (MDBK) as they reduced their viability by 3–17%. A change in the distribution of the cell cycle phases in the non-infected cell population treated with EPSs was observed. The analysis demonstrated an increase in the number of cells in the S phase by 47% when using EPSs 15a and a decrease in the number of cells in the G1 phase by 20–27% when treated with the EPSs 15a, 33a, and 19s. The use of EPSs did not led to the normalization of the life cycle of HAdV-5 infected cells to the level of non-infected cells. The EPSs showed low virucidal activity and reduced the HAdV-5 infectivity to 85%. Among the studied exopolysaccharides, anti-adenovirus activity was found for EPS 26a that is produced by *Lactobacillus* spp. strain. The treatment of cells with the EPS following virus adsorption completely (100%) suppressed the formation and release of HAdV-5 infectious. *Conclusions:* EPS 26a possessed distinct anti-HAdV-5 activity and the obtained data demonstrate the potential of using exopolysaccharides as anti-adenoviral agents.

Keywords: exopolysaccharides; lactic acid bacteria; human adenovirus type 5; antiviral activity; cell cycle

1. Introduction

Despite successes of vaccination, chemoprevention, and chemotherapy of human respiratory viral infections, these diseases still are one of the leading causes of human infectious disorders. Adenoviruses cause keratoconjunctivitis, as well as respiratory, urogenital and intestinal tract infectious diseases. In addition, adenoviruses may persist in the lymphoid tissue of the tonsils and adenoids for a long time, causing upper respiratory tract infections in adults [1,2].

Various compounds have been found to be effective against adenoviruses. Anti-adenoviral activity was shown in vitro for nucleotide analogs [3,4]. Ribavirin, which affects many DNA and RNA-containing viruses, was found to be effective, partially effective, or not effective against adenoviral infection. Ganciclovir, which is efficient against cytomegalovirus infection, is effective against adenoviruses both in vitro and in vivo [5]. Cidofovir, which is characterized by a broad spectrum of antiviral activity, is used for the treatment of severe adenoviral infections [6]. Ribavirin, ganciclovir, and cidofovir are more or less successfully used for the treatment of severe human adenoviral pathologies, including hepatitis, cystitis, and pneumonia in immunocompromised organ transplant recipients [7,8]. At the same time, apparent adverse effects and the ability of adenoviruses to form resistant strains limit the use of these drugs [9]. Some chemically distinct compounds, including lipids, acridones, and imidazoquinolinamines, as well as other analogs of nucleosides, also show anti-adenoviral activity. Virus reproduction in cell cultures may be inhibited by high concentrations of green tea catechins [10]. Interferon drugs used to treat respiratory infections are most useful for prevention and cannot be considered as the primary medications for the treatment of severe infection. As adenoviruses have effective mechanisms that suppress the interferon-induced antiviral cascade, they are resistant to the action of interferon and its inducers [11].

Therefore, the development of new antiviral drugs that would be effective against adenoviruses without adverse effects, for a wide range of patients, including long-term users, is very urgent.

Currently, the use of probiotic antagonist microorganisms and their metabolic products represents a promising approach for the treatment of viral diseases [12]. Lactic acid bacteria (LAB), which can be found in the microbiota of the mucous membranes of the nose and mouth, and the gastrointestinal and urinary tracts, have a positive effect on these ecosystems as they stimulate the immune system and increase resistance to infections of bacterial and viral origin. LAB are the sources of multiple biologically active substances that vary in chemical structure and action spectrum [13]. During metabolic processes, lactic acid bacteria produce vital substances, including vitamins, amino acids, enzymes, fatty acids, exopolysaccharides, lactic acid, bacteriocins, and hydrogen peroxide, and significantly improve the intestinal absorption of micro- and macro-elements essential for the organism. It was also shown that exopolysaccharides that are secreted during the cultivation of LAB, in addition to their probiotic activity, can act selectively on pathogenic microbes and viruses without significant disturbances of the microbiocenosis and the development of inflammatory processes that occur during the use of broad-spectrum antibiotics and chemical antiviral agents [14]. As a result, exopolysaccharides can be used as a base for the production of harmless, non-toxic and acellular probiotic products and drugs that have a targeted therapeutic effect.

The present study aimed to investigate the antiviral activity of exopolysaccharides produced by lactic acid bacteria of the genera *Pediococcus*, *Leuconostoc* and *Lactobacillus* against human adenovirus type 5.

2. Materials and Methods

2.1. Virus and Cell Culture

In this study MDBK cells were obtained from the tissue culture collection of the Institute of Virology of the Bulgarian Academy of Sciences (Sofia, Bulgaria) and HAdV-5 was obtained from the collection of the Institute of Microbiology of the Budapest University of Medical Sciences (Budapest, Hungary) and propagated in HEp-2 (ATCC CCL-23) cells.

MDBK cells were maintained in sterile plastic falcon ® (Sarstedt AG & Co. KG, Nümbrecht, Germany) in a growth medium composed of 45% DMEM (Sigma-Aldrich, St. Louis, MO, USA), 45% RPMI 1640 (Sigma-Aldrich, St. Louis, MO, USA) and 10% fetal bovine serum (FBS, Sigma-Aldrich, St. Louis, MO, USA) heat inactivated at 56 °C with antibiotics penicillin (Sigma-Aldrich, St. Louis, MO, USA) and streptomycin (100 µg/mL) (Sigma-Aldrich, St. Louis, MO, USA).

Cultivation, purification, and preservation of HAdV-5 were performed according to the standard method [15]. The infectious titer of the virus in MDBK cell culture was 7.0×10^7 PFU/mL.

2.2. Tested Substances

Exopolysaccharides (EPSs) produced by lactic acid bacteria of the genera *Pediococcus, Leuconostoc* and *Lactobacillus* were extracted, purified and accumulated by the researchers from the Department of Physiology of Industrial Microorganisms at the Zabolotny Institute of Microbiology and Virology National Academy of Sciences of Ukraine (Table 1) [16,17]. Ribavirin (Rib) (Sigma-Aldrich, St. Louis, MO, USA) was used as a reference compound.

Table 1. Sources used to extract exopolysaccharides (EPSs) and genera of lactic acid bacteria (LAB) producing respective EPS.

EPS	Source of Extracted EPS	Genus of Lactic Acid Bacteria
6a	pickled apples	*Pediococcus* sp.
48a	pickled apples	*Leuconostoc* sp.
2t	pickled tomato juice	*Leuconostoc* sp.
19s	sauerkraut	*Leuconostoc* sp.
6s	sauerkraut	*Leuconostoc* sp.
26a	pickled apples	*Lactobacillus* sp.

2.3. Cytotoxicity Assays

MTT-assay was used for the analysis of cell viability [18]. After 24 h of growth in growth medium, monolayers of MDBK cells in 96-multiwell plates were incubated with EPS at the concentrations of 375, 750 and 1500 µg/mL. Control cells were incubated with fresh medium lacking EPS for 72 h. A total of 20 µL of MTT solution 3-(4,5-dimethylthiazol-2-yl)-2,5-diphenyl tetrazolium bromide (Sigma-Aldrich, St. Louis, MO, USA) was added into wells and cells were incubated at 37 °C and 5% CO_2 for 3–4 h, then the medium was removed and 150 µL of 96% ethanol was added. The plates were read using a Multiskan FC (Thermo Scientific, Waltham, MA, USA) with a 538-nm test wavelength.

Percentage decrease of cell viability under the condition of EPS action was calculated by the following formula:

$$\% \text{ decrease of cell viability} = 100 - (A/B \times 100) \quad (1)$$

where A is the mean optical density of the studied samples at a certain concentration, and B is the mean optical density of the control cell samples.

EPS concentration at which cell viability was inhibited by 50% (CC_{50}) was estimated in comparison to the control cells not treated with EPS.

2.4. Cell Cycle Analysis by Flow Cytometry

MDBK cells infected with adenovirus (treated and not treated with the EPSs) were fixed in 96% ice-cold ethanol for 1 h, resuspended in 500 mL solution of phosphate-buffered saline (Sigma-Aldrich, St. Louis, MO, USA) that contained RNAse (100 µg/mL) (AppliChem GmbH, Darmstadt, Germany) and propidium iodide (PI) (50 µg/mL) (Sigma-Aldrich, St. Louis, MO, USA), and incubated at room temperate in a dark place for 1 h [19]. The cell fluorescence intensity was measured by a flow cytometer (Beckman Coulter Epics LX, Minneapolis, MN, USA) with a laser wavelength of 488 nm. A total of 20,000 cells were sorted per sample. Cell cycle profiles were analyzed with the program Flowing Software, v. 2.5 (Cell Imaging Core, Finland).

2.5. Antiviral Assay

To investigate the best order of EPSs' antiviral effects, three experimental procedures were used as follows:

2.5.1. Pre-Treatment of Cells with EPSs

To MDBK cells were added 100 μL of EPSs at the concentrations of 20, 100 and 500 μg/mL, which were then incubated at 37 °C for 24 h. Then, cells were infected with HAdV-5 (the multiplicity of the infection (MOI) of 7 PFU per cell). After 1.5 h, the virus-containing medium was removed, and 200 μL of serum-free medium was added.

2.5.2. Co-Incubation of EPSs and HAdV-5

Adenovirus (MOI 70 PFU/cell) was mixed with an equal volume of EPS at a concentration of 1500 μg/mL and incubated at 37 °C for 3 h. The MDBK cell monolayer was infected with 50 μL per well of suspension of EPS-HAdV-5 of the appropriate dilution. Following the virus adsorption that was carried out at 37 °C for 1.5 h, the virus-containing material was removed, and 200 μL of serum-free medium was added.

2.5.3. EPSs Were Added Post-Infection

The MDBK cells were first infected with HAdV-5 at 50 μL/well (MOI 3.5 PFU/cell), and the virus was adsorbed at 37 °C for 1.5 h. Then, the virus was removed, and the growth medium with the appropriate EPSs concentration was added (20, 100 and 500 μg/mL).

Plates with cells were kept at 5% CO_2 at 37 °C until a visible cytopathic effect of adenovirus appeared (3–5 days), and the virus material was selected for further investigation of the virus titer. Non-treated cells and cells treated with HAdV-5 served as controls.

2.6. Virus Titration

The titer of the virus was determined by the plaque method, based on the formation of necrotic sites in the infected cells due to the reproduction of the virus. Cells were grown in a 24-well plate (TPP, Trasadingen, Switzerland) to form a 100% monolayer and were infected with serial ten-fold diluted lysates of cells previously infected with adenovirus (untreated or treated with different concentrations of EPSs) at 0.3 mL per well and incubated for 1.5 h at 37 °C at 5% CO_2. After adsorption of the virus, the medium was removed, and the cells were covered with 1% methylcellulose (Sigma-Aldrich, St. Louis, MO, USA), DMEM medium (Sigma-Aldrich, St. Louis, MO, USA) and 2% fetal bovine serum (Sigma-Aldrich, St. Louis, MO, USA). Cells were incubated at 37 °C at 5% CO_2 for 5 days. Next, the cover was removed and 200 μL of 0.2% crystal violet (Sigma-Aldrich, St. Louis, MO, USA) in 20% ethanol was added to the cell monolayer [20,21]. The titer of the virus was determined by the highest dilution of the virus in which the virus-induced plaques were formed according to the formula:

$$\text{Virus titer PFU/mL} = A/(B \times C) \quad (2)$$

where A is the number of plaques, B is the dilution of the virus, and C is the volume of the inoculum.

The antiviral activity of EPSs was determined using the following formula:

$$\%\ \text{inhibition} = (1 - \text{Virus titer (experiment)/virus titer (control)}) \times 100\% \quad (3)$$

A decrease in the infectious titer of the virus by 2 lg or more (or 99% or more), compared with the control, indicates significant activity of the compound against the virus, 97–99% demonstrates a moderate effect and less than 97% shows a relative activity [22].

2.7. Statistical Analysis

Statistical data processing was performed according to standard approaches for calculating statistical errors (standard deviation) using Microsoft Excel 2010. The results were expressed as mean ± S.D. for three independent experiments. The Student's *t*-test (unpaired, two-sided *t*-test) was used to evaluate the difference between the test sample and control. A p value of <0.05 was considered statistically significant.

3. Results

3.1. The Effect of Lactic Acid Bacteria Exopolysaccarides on Viability and Mitotic Activity of MDBK Cells

The issue of directed inhibition of the reproduction of infectious disease pathogens requires a search for medicines that are characterized by low toxicity and a broad spectrum of antiviral activity. As viruses are intracellular parasites, selective suppression of virus reproduction without adverse effect on the viability of host cells is one of the requirements for antiviral inhibitors.

MTT analysis is one of the most simple and available methods for the estimation of cytotoxicity. The technique enables the identification of the negative impact of EPSs on the viability of cells and the functional activity of mitochondria (Figure 1).

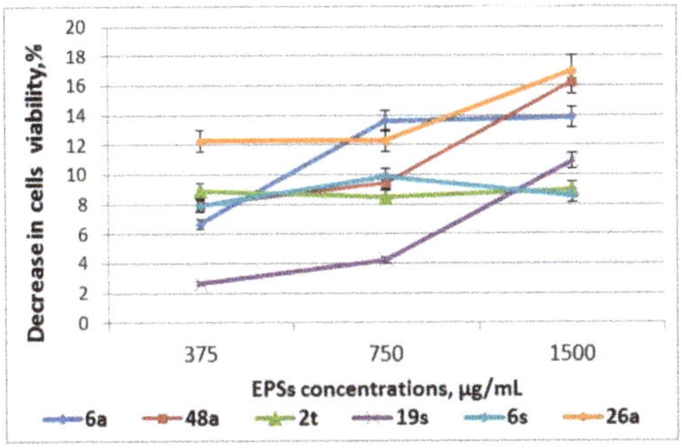

Figure 1. Cytotoxicity of exopolysaccharides in MDBK cells. Serial three-fold dilutions of EPSs in DMEM-RPMI medium were added onto the monolayer of MDBK in a 96-well plate for 72 h at 37 °C. Cell viability effect was determined by MTT assay. Values represent the mean ± S.D. for three independent experiments.

It was found that EPSs at a concentration of 375–1500 µg/mL were not toxic for MDBK cells, as they suppressed their viability only by 3–17%, whereas the CC_{50} value was significantly higher than 1500 µg/mL. The CC_{50} value for referent compound Ribavirin was 400 µg/mL.

As toxic compounds often cause the termination of cell growth and proliferation, the effect of EPSs on the MDBK cell populations was studied. Cells were fixed and dyed with fluorochrome propidium iodide and analyzed using flow cytometry. The approach allowed the estimation of the distribution of cells by their structure and cell cycle phases, as well as the identification of apoptotic cells, as the propidium iodide signal is directly proportional to DNA content.

As can be seen from cell cycle profiles (Figure 2A) based on the distribution of cells according to the structure and cell cycle phase, the histograms of EPS-treated and control MDBK cells are similar but not identical. It was revealed that after 48 h of growth, 50% of control MDBK cells remained in the G1 phase, 16% were in the S phase, and 13% were in the G2/M phases (Figure 2B).

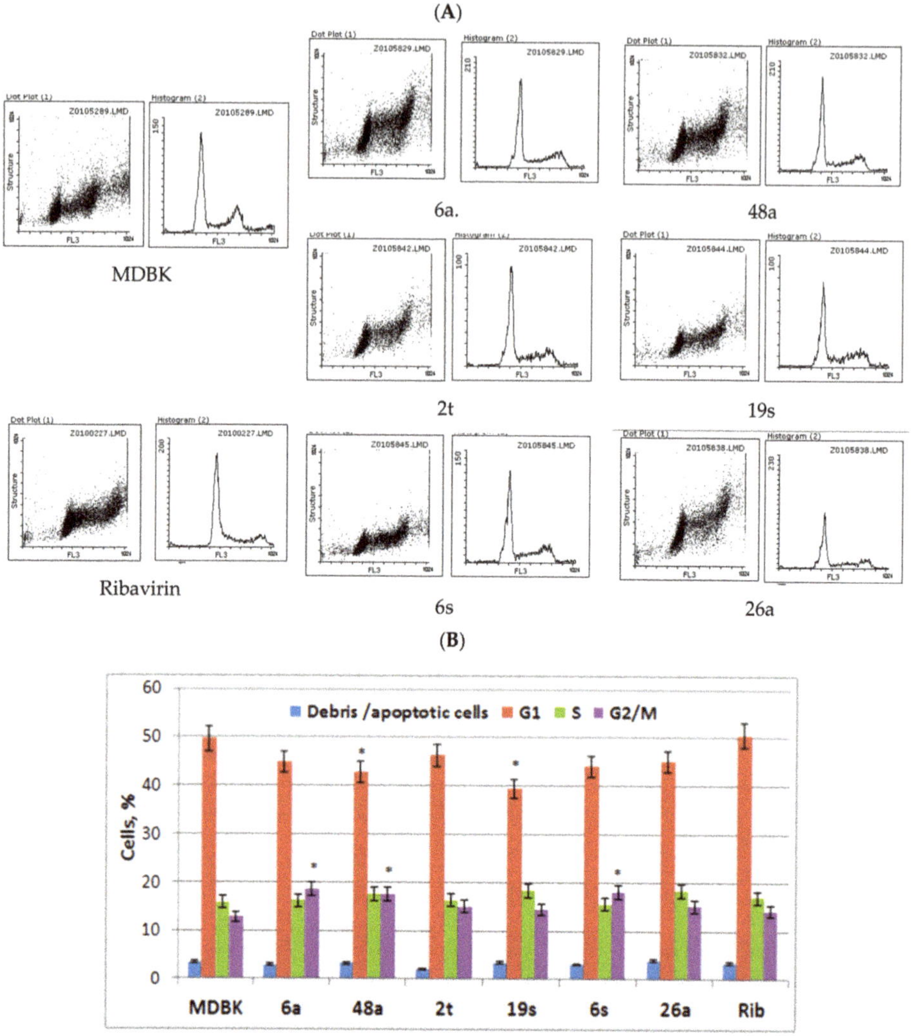

Figure 2. Influence of the EPSs on the cell cycle of the MDBK cells. (**A**) Cell cycle profiles of the control cells and EPS-treated cells (concentration of exopolysaccharides and ribavirin are 1500 and 125 μg/mL, respectively). (**B**) Cell cycle features after treatment with the EPSs were measured by flow cytometry following cell fixation and propidium iodide staining. Cell cycle profiles were analyzed with the Flowing Software, version 2.5. Results corresponding to the percentage of cells in G1, S, and G2/M phases of three independent experiments are presented as mean ± S.D. * Significant difference between test sample and control cells ($p < 0.05$).

Under the conditions of the compound treatment, the distribution of cells in G1 and G2/M phases was similar to control cells. However, compared to control cells, EPSs 48a and 19s decreased the number of cells in the G1 phase up to 16%, whereas EPSs 6a, 48a, and 6s increased the number of cells in the G2/M phase by 11–42%.

3.2. Anti-Adenoviral Activity of EPSs

The anti-HAdV-5 activity of EPSs (in non-toxic concentrations) was confirmed by measuring virus yield synthesized de novo using a plaque reduction assay.

Analysis of the antiviral activity of EPSs added to MDBK cells 24 h before adenovirus infection demonstrated that only EPSs 48a, 26a and 6s showed low antiviral activity, reducing virus reproduction by 23–67% (Figure 3), indicating the inefficiency of EPS use according to the suggested treatment approach.

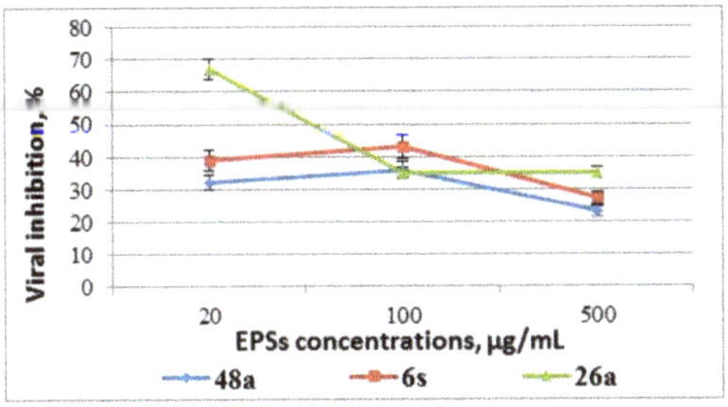

Figure 3. Effect of EPSs on infectivity of adenoviral offspring: the results of the analysis of the EPS-mediated antiviral effect for pre-treatment of cells with EPSs. Results are presented as percentage of infectious virus titer reduction and are the mean of three independent experiments.

It was found that EPS showed weak virucidal activity decreasing the infectious titer of HAdV-5 by 3–85%, whereas incubation of the virus with EPS 6a increased HAdV-5 reproduction by 15% (Figure 4).

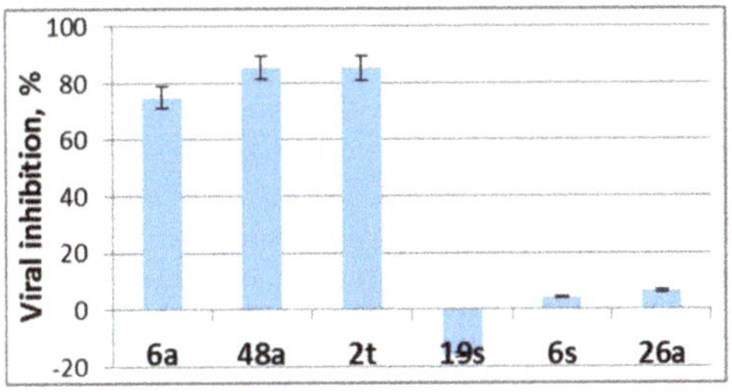

Figure 4. Influence of EPSs on the formation of infectious progeny of adenovirus. The results of the analysis of the EPS-mediated antiviral effect for co-incubation of EPSs (concentration 1500 µg/mL) and HAdV-5. Results are presented as percentage of infectious virus titer reduction and are the mean of three independent experiments.

Using EPSs at late stages of adenovirus reproduction and immediately after virus adsorption, it was found that only EPS 26a shows apparent anti-HAdV-5 activity. At the concentrations of 20 and 100 µg/mL, the EPS absolutely blocked the synthesis of viral progeny (Figure 5). Other EPSs used in the analyzed concentrations reduced the infectious titer of the virus by 18–93%. The use of Ribavirin at concentrations of 32–125 µg/mL after infection of the cells with adenovirus resulted in a decrease in HAdV-5 reproduction by 96.3–99.8% (data not shown).

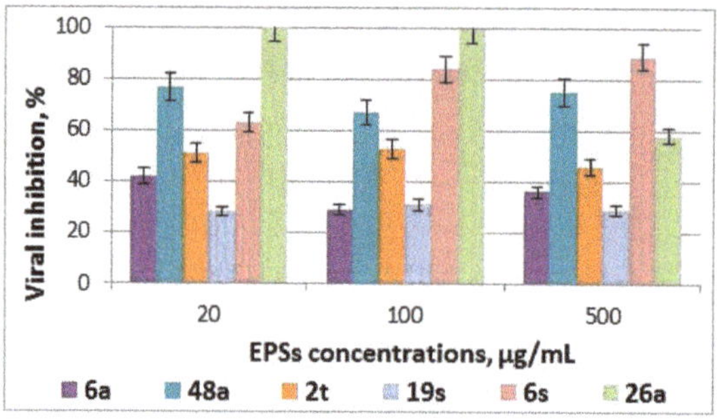

Figure 5. Effect of EPSs on adenovirus reproduction: the results of the analysis of the antiviral activity of EPSs added after infection. Results are presented as percentage of infectious virus titer reduction and are the mean of three independent experiments.

Virus infection frequently results in the disturbance of key cellular processes within the host cell. The subversion of cell cycle pathways is a well-established mechanism by which viruses create the most suitable environment for their replication [23]. Notably, the induction of the S-phase is either mandatory or at least advantageous for lytic replication of a number of viruses. Adenoviral infection has been reported to have effects on the cell cycle. It is well-known that adenoviral E1 gene products interact with pRb (retinoblastoma protein), causing the release of E2F transcription factor, which potentiates transition from the G1 to the S phase, in which productivity is greatest. HAdV infection of a range of epithelial cell lines, including a primary cell line, causes G2 phase synchronization and cell cycle arrest [24,25]. This synchronization in the G2 phase may be a significant factor contributing to the cell-size increase [25]. Therefore, the influence of EPSs on the cell cycle under the conditions of adenovirus infection was analyzed using flow cytometric analysis.

Significant changes in the cell cycle of cells infected with HAdV-5 compared to non-infected cells were revealed. In particular, the number of cells in the G1 phase decreased by 67%, whereas the number of cells in the S phase is doubled (Figure 6). The reduction of the cell population in G1 phases demonstrated the suppression of the transition of cells through the mitotic phase. As infected cells enter the S phase and the G2/M phase is blocked, cells produce viral DNA, late viral proteins and virions. Further, these cells are destroyed and detach from the monolayer.

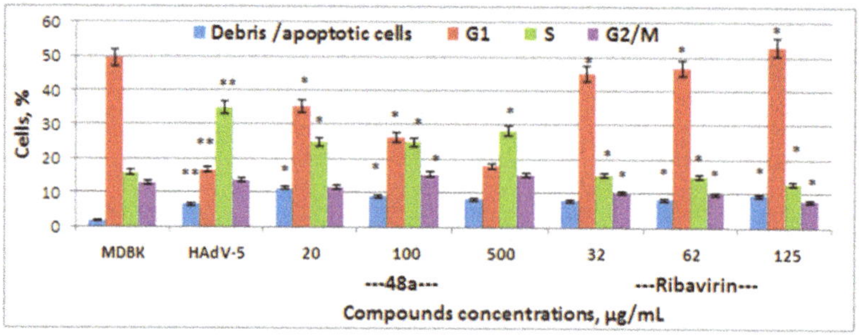

Figure 6. Influence of the EPSs on the cell cycle of the MDBK in the presence of adenovirus infection. The cells' fluorescence intensity was measured by a flow cytometer (Beckman Coulter Epics LX, MN, USA) with laser wavelength 488 nm. Cell cycle profiles were analyzed with the program Flowing Software, version 2.5. Results corresponding to the percentage of cells in the G1, S, and G2/M phases of three independent experiments are presented as mean ± S.D. * Significant difference between test sample and control of infected cells ($p < 0.05$). ** Significant difference between a control of infected cells and control cells ($p < 0.05$).

It was found that after the treatment of cells infected with adenovirus using exopolysaccharides, the distribution of cells in cell cycle phases was similar to the distribution of cells infected with adenovirus, demonstrating the inefficiency of the exopolysaccharide treatment (data not shown). A decrease in the number of cells in the S phase by 5–33% compared with the distribution of infected cells was observed. However, there was no increase in the number of cells in the G1 phase, indicating continued blocking of the mitotic phase of the cell cycle due to viral infection. Only the use of EPS 48a at a concentration of 100 and 20 μg/mL resulted in a significant increase in the number of cells in the G1 phase (1.5–2 times) compared with infected cells, and a decrease in the number of cells in the synthetic phase by 18–29%, indicating normalization of the cell cycle of infected cells to the level of uninfected cells (Figure 6).

4. Discussion

In recent years, there has been a tendency to use LAB exopolysaccharides for the treatment of infections of the respiratory tract, gastrointestinal tract, and urinary system, as well as cancer, allergic diseases, and viral infections [26]. However, despite the wide range of applications of lactic acid bacteria exopolysaccharides, their role in living organisms and their biological activities are not fully understood. The production of exopolysaccharides (EPS) by lactic acid bacteria (LAB) has been intensively studied, and a significant amount of data describing their composition, structure, and properties have been accumulated. EPS producing strains were found among representatives of the genera *Streptococcus, Lactococcus, Lactobacillus, Leuconostoc, Pediococcus,* and *Weissella*. LAB exopolysaccharides have unique physical and rheological properties. As a result, they are used in the food industry as binding, stabilizing, and gel-forming agents, specifically in the production of dairy products. In recent years, much attention has been paid to the study of the biological activity of EPSs. In particular, it was shown that they have immunostimulating, antitumor, and antioxidant qualities. Since the biological activity of EPSs is strain-specific, the search for new strain-producers among LAB representatives found in the natural microbiota of fermented products is of great interest. Strains producing EPSs, especially in high amounts, are important for improving the rheological properties of the product and may possess possible health-improving effects for the human body. Previously, searches for LAB strains producing exopolysaccharides were performed. The isolates of LAB present in traditional fermented milk products, fermented fruits and vegetables were analyzed. Most EPS producers were found among representatives of the genera *Lactobacillus, Leuconostoc* and *Pediococcus* isolated from pickled apples, pickled tomato juice, and sauerkraut. Therefore, the biological activity of these EPSs was analyzed in the current work. In the preclinical study of potential drugs, the first step is associated with the assessment of the compound's toxicity for cell culture (namely, the study of the effect of different concentrations on the structural and functional properties of the cells). It should be noted that most toxic agents act on the cell by interfering with the molecular mechanisms of homeostasis. This action can be expressed in a whole set of effects, which include changes in the fundamental cellular reactions, leading to destructive effects. We have studied the impact of EPSs extracted from lactic acid bacteria of the genera *Pediococcus, Leuconostoc* and *Lactobacillus* on the growth and division of MDBK cells sensitive to adenovirus. It was identified that EPSs in the studied concentrations are not toxic to MDBK cells, since they reduce cell viability only up to 17%. Also, the analysis of the effect of the highest EPS concentration on the cell cycle of MDBK cells showed the absence of significant changes in the distribution of the cell population in the G1, S and G2/M phases of the cycle. The obtained data allowed the use of all EPSs for the study of their antiviral potential. It is known that bacterial exopolysaccharides show significant antiviral activity due to the degradation of the viral particles, a decrease in the titer of viruses, the blocking of viral DNA replication, and the release of the infectious virus particle. However, the antiviral potential of these drugs has not been studied sufficiently. As a result, to investigate and exhibit EPS-mediated anti-adenoviral activity and to determine the stage of viral reproduction inhibited by EPS, various EPS treatment schemes were used in the work. Based on three different treatments, the results suggested that EPSs have a specific inhibitory effect on HAdV-5. The EPSs showed low virucidal activity and reduced HAdV-5 infectivity up to 85%. In most cases, neither pre-treatment resulted in a significant inactivation of virion infectivity. The inhibitory effects were observed only when EPSs were added to cells at the end of the virus adsorption period. However, only EPS 26a (produced by *Lactobacillus* sp.) reduced the titer of the virus obtained de novo and inhibited HAdV-5 plaque formation by 100%.

Currently, several possible mechanisms of the influence of lactic acid bacteria and their metabolites on the development of viral infection have been identified: i) inhibition of virus adsorption and penetration into cells as a result of direct bacterium/metabolite-virus interaction; ii) inhibition of late stages of viral reproduction and reduction of their infectivity; and, iii) stimulation of the immune system [26]. As a result, it was shown that probiotics can "capture" the virus of vesicular stomatitis (VSV) by direct interaction between LAB cells (*L. paracasei A14, L. paracasei F19, L. paracasei/rhamnosus Q8, L. plantarum M1.1* and *L. reuteri DSM12246*) and the lipid envelope of the VSV, which leads to blocking of the virus adsorption on the cell. Similar data were shown for *E. faecium NCIMB 10415* against influenza viruses and *L. gasseri CMUL57* isolated from vaginal microbiota against the herpes simplex virus type 2 (HSV-2). The probiotics of lactic acid bacteria *Lactobacillus* and their exopolysaccharides can stimulate the synthesis and accumulation of interleukin 12 to enhance the activity of natural killer cells and the synthesis of IgA in the spleen. Such activation of Th1 immune responses and the production of IgA determine their action against influenza [27]. In addition to direct interaction between viruses and LAB, bacteria synthesize some metabolites with antiviral activity. As a result, hydrogen peroxide, which is produced by *Lactobacillus* sp., plays an essential role as a natural microbocide within the vaginal ecosystem and is toxic to human immunodeficiency virus type 1 (HIV-1) and HSV-2. Lactic acid, which is the final product of carbohydrate metabolism and is synthesized by all types of lactobacilli, is essential for maintaining the required pH of the genital organs, since it is known that the acidic pH of the environment inactivates HIV, and HSV-1 and -2. It has been revealed that lactobacilli can produce compounds that inhibit replication of the viruses. The *L. brevis* cell wall inhibits the replication of HSV-2 DNA in cell culture, while the acidic products of the *Lactobacillus* metabolism inhibit the activation of T-lymphocytes, leading to a decrease in the sensitivity of lymphocytes to HIV infection, which is especially important for mixed HIV–HSV infections [28]. It has been established that some types of bacteriocins and exopolysaccharides have an apparent virucidal effect on influenza, HSV-1 and -2, HIV and Newcastle disease.

The characteristic changes in DNA synthesis and content induced by HAdV-5 infection allow the use of flow cytometry to detect not only viral infection but also potential antiviral activities [25]. The influence of the EPSs on the cell cycle under a condition of adenovirus infection was studied using flow cytometric analysis of propidium iodide-stained cells. The use of EPSs did not lead to the normalization of the life cycle of HAdV-5 infected cells to the level of non-infected cells, as the number of cells in the S phase was not decreased significantly (except EPS 48a) and there was no transition of cells into the G1 phase, which indicates the blocking of the mitosis in infected cells.

Taken together, our data suggested that exopolysaccharides produced by LAB strains exhibited anti-HAdV-5 activity in vitro. Among the six used strains, one LAB strain (*Lactobacillus* sp.), which produced EPS 26a suppressing the yield of virus particles, was selected. Furthermore, this strain is interesting as potential probiotic or starter, whereas the in-depth investigation of the functional and technological properties, EPSs monosaccharide composition and structure are currently studied.

5. Conclusions

In summary, the EPS 26a produced by *Lactobacillus* sp. possessed significant anti-HAdV-5 activity, based on the obstruction of HAdV-5 reproduction, inducing the formation of non-infectious virus progeny. Thus, this LAB strain is a promising producer of EPS with antiviral activity against HAdV-5. However, further investigation is needed to explore the antiviral mechanism of such an EPS in detail.

Author Contributions: Conceptualization, L.B. and Y.P.; Funding acquisition, L.B.; Investigation, L.B., Y.P., O.P.; Methodology, S.Z. and L.B; Resources, S.Z. and L.B.; Visualization, L.B.; Writing-original draft, L.B.; Writing—review & editing, O.P. and S.Z.

Funding: This research was funded by the State Fund for Fundamental Research of Ukraine (grant number F83).

Acknowledgments: We thank Vasyliuk O.M. and Garmasheva I.L. from the department of physiology of industrial microorganisms of the Danylo Zabolotny Institute of Microbiology and Virology NASU for the provided exopolysaccharides used in the study.

Conflicts of Interest: The authors declare no conflict of interest.

References

1. Ghebremedhin, B. Human adenovirus: Viral pathogen with increasing importance. *Eur. J. Microbiol. Immunol.* **2014**, *4*, 26–33. [CrossRef] [PubMed]
2. Robinson, C.M.; Singh, G.; Lee, J.Y.; Dehghan, S.; Rajaiya, J.; Liu, E.B.; Yousuf, M.A.; Betensky, R.A.; Jones, M.S.; Dyer, D.W.; et al. Molecular evolution of human adenoviruses. *Sci. Rep.* **2013**, *3*, 1812–1817. [CrossRef] [PubMed]
3. De Clercq, E. Curious (old and new) antiviral nucleoside analogues with intriguing therapeutic potential. *Med. Chem.* **2015**, *22*, 3866–3880. [CrossRef]
4. Zarubaev, V.V.; Slita, A.V.; Sirotkin, A.K.; Nebolsin, E.V.; Kiselev, O.I. Experimental Study of Ingavirin® Antiviral Activity Against Human Adenovirus. *Antibiotiki i khimioterapiia* **2010**, *55*, 19–24. [PubMed]
5. Ying, B.; Tollefson, A.E.; Spencer, J.F.; Balakrishnan, L.; Dewhurst, S.; Capella, C.; Buller, R.M.R.; Toth, K.; Wold, W.S.M. Ganciclovir inhibits human adenovirus replication and pathogenicity in permissive immunosuppressive Syrian hamsters. *Antimicrob. Agents Chemother.* **2014**, *58*, 7171–7181. [CrossRef] [PubMed]
6. Safrin, S.; Cherrington, J.; Joffe, H.S. Cidofovir. Review of current and potential clinical uses. *Adv. Exp. Med. Biol.* **1999**, *458*, 111–120. [PubMed]
7. De Clercq, E.; Li, E.G. Approved Antiviral Drugs over the Past 50 Years. *Clin. Microbiol. Rev.* **2016**, *29*, 695–747. [CrossRef] [PubMed]
8. Morfin, F.; Dupuis-Girod, S.; Frobert, E.; Mundweiler, S.; Carrington, D.; Sedlacek, P.; Bierings, M.; Cetkovsky, P.; Kroes, A.C.; van Tol, M.J.; et al. Differential susceptibility of adenovirus clinical isolates to cidofovir and ribavirin is not related to species alone. *Antivir. Ther.* **2009**, *14*, 55–61.
9. Waye, M.M.Y.; Sing, C.W. Anti-Viral Drugs for Human Adenoviruses. *Pharmaceuticals* **2010**, *3*, 3343–3354. [CrossRef]
10. Weber, J.M.; Ruzindana-Umunyana, A.; Imbeault, L.; Sircar, S. Inhibition of adenovirus infection and adenain by green tea catechins. *Antiviral Res.* **2003**, *58*, 167–173. [CrossRef]
11. Zhang, Y.; Schneider, R.J. Adenovirus inhibition of cellular protein synthesis and the specific translation of late viral mRNAs. *Semin. Virol.* **1993**, *4*, 229–236. [CrossRef]
12. Ryan, P.M.; Ross, R.P.; Fitzgerald, G.F.; Caplice, N.M.; Stanton, C. Sugarcoated: Exopolysaccharide producing lactic acid bacteria for food and human health applications. *Food Func.* **2015**, *6*, 679–693. [CrossRef]
13. Kassaa, I.; Hober, D.; Hamze, M.; Chihib, N.E.; Drider, D. Antiviral Potential of Lactic Acid Bacteria and Their Bacteriocins. *Probiotics Antimicro.* **2014**, *6*, 177–185. [CrossRef] [PubMed]
14. Gugliandolo, C.; Spanò, A.; Maugeri, T.L.; Poli, A.; Arena, A.; Nicolaus, B. Role of Bacterial Exopolysaccharides as Agents in Counteracting Immune Disorders Induced by Herpes Virus. *Microorganisms* **2015**, *3*, 464–483. [CrossRef] [PubMed]
15. Green, M.; Loewenstein, P.M. Human adenoviruses: Propagation, purification, quantification, and storage. *Curr. Protoc. Microbiol.* **2006**, 14C.1.1–14C.1.19. [CrossRef]
16. Garmasheva, I. Isolation and characterization of lactic acid bacteria from Ukrainian traditional dairy products. *AIMS Microbiol.* **2016**, *2*, 372–387.
17. Garmasheva, I.L.; Kovalenko, N.K.; Vasyluk, O.M.; Oleschenko, L.T. Exopolysaccharides Production By Lactic Acid Bacteria Strains Isolated From Fernmented Products. *Microbiology&Biotechnology* **2017**, *4*, 76–84. [CrossRef]
18. Mosmann, T. Rapid colorimetric assay for cellular growth and surviral: Application to proliferation and cytotoxicity assays. *J. Immunol. Methods* **1983**, *65*, 55–63. [CrossRef]

19. Kim, K.H.; Sederstrom, J.M. Assaying cell cycle status using flow cytometry. *Curr Protoc Mol Biol.* **2015**, *111*, 28.6.1–28.6.11. [CrossRef]
20. Das, A.; Trousdale, M.D.; Ren, S.; Lien, E.J. Inhibition of herpes simplex virus type 1 and adenovirus type 5 by heterocyclic Schiff bases of aminohydroxyguanidine tosylate. *Antivir. Res.* **1999**, *44*, 201–208. [CrossRef]
21. Cromeans, T.L.; Lub, X.; Erdman, D.D.; Humphreyc, C.D.; Hill, V.R. Development of plaque assays for adenoviruses 40 and 41. *J. Virol. Methods.* **2008**, *151*, 140–145. [CrossRef] [PubMed]
22. Kohn, L.K.; Foglio, M.A.; Rodrigues, R.A.; Sousa, I.M.; Martini, M.C.; Padilla, M.A.; de Lima, N.; Arns, C.W. In Vitro Antiviral Activities of Extracts of Plants of The Brazilian Cerrado against the Avian Metapneumovirus (aMPV). *Braz. J. Poultry Sci.* **2015**, *17*, 275–280. [CrossRef]
23. Trapp-Fragnet, L.; Bencherit, D.; Chabanne-Vautherot, D.; Vern, Y.L.; Remy, S.; Boutet-Robinet, E.; Mirey, G.; Vautherot, K.F.; Denesvre, C. Cell Cycle Modulation by Marek's Disease Virus: The Tegument Protein VP22 Triggers S-Phase Arrest and DNA Damage in Proliferating Cells. *PLOS ONE* **2014**, *9*, 1–14. [CrossRef] [PubMed]
24. Grand, R.J.; Ibrahim, A.P.; Taylor, A.M.; Milner, A.E.; Gregory, C.D.; Gallimore, P.H.; Turnell, A.S. Human Cells Arrest in S Phase in Response to Adenovirus 12 E1A. *Virology* **1998**, *244*, 330–342. [CrossRef] [PubMed]
25. Sandhu, K.; Al-Rubeai, M. Monitoring of the Adenovirus Production Process by Flow Cytometry. *Biotechnol Prog.* **2008**, *24*, 250–260. [CrossRef] [PubMed]
26. Yang, Y.; Song, H.; Wang, L.; Dong, W.; Yang, Z.; Yuan, P.; Wang, K.; Song, Z. Antiviral Effects of a Probiotic Metabolic Products against Transmissible Gastroenteritis Coronavirus. *J Prob Health.* **2017**, *5*, 184. [CrossRef]
27. Jung, Y.J.; Lee, Y.T.; Ngo, V.L.; Cho, Y.H.; Ko, E.J.; Hong, S.M.; Kim, K.H.; Jang, J.H.; Oh, J.S.; Park, M.K.; et al. Heat-killed *Lactobacillus casei* confers broad protection against influenza A virus primary infection and develops heterosubtypic immunity against future secondary infection. *Sci. Rep.* **2017**, *7*, 17360. [CrossRef]
28. Martín, V.; Maldonado, A.; Fernández, L.; Rodríguez, J.M.; Connor, R.I. Inhibition of Human Immunodeficiency Virus Type 1 by Lactic Acid Bacteria from Human Breastmilk. *Breastfeed Med.* **2010**, *5*, 153–158. [CrossRef]

medicina

MDPI

Article

A Retrospective Study about the Impact of Switching from Nested PCR to Multiplex Real-Time PCR on the Distribution of the Human Papillomavirus (HPV) Genotypes

Raffaele Del Prete [1,2], Luigi Ronga [2], Grazia Addati [1], Raffaella Magrone [1], Angela Abbasciano [1], Domenico Di Carlo [3,4] and Luigi Santacroce [2,5,*]

1 Section of Microbiology, Interdisciplinary Department of Medicine (DIM), School of Medicine, University of Bari "Aldo Moro", 70124 Bari, Italy
2 UOC Microbiology and Virology, Azienda Ospedaliera-Universitaria Policlinico of Bari, 70124 Bari, Italy
3 Pediatric Clinical Research Center "Romeo and Erica Invernizzi", University of Milan, 20157 Milan, Italy
4 Department of Biology and Biotechnology, University of Pavia, 27100 Pavia, Italy
5 Ionian Department, University of Bari "Aldo Moro", 70100 Bari, Italy
* Correspondence: luigi.santacroce@uniba.it; Tel./Fax: +39-080-5478496

Received: 19 June 2019; Accepted: 26 July 2019; Published: 30 July 2019

Abstract: Background and objectives: Human papillomavirus (HPV) is the most prevalent etiological agent of viral sexually-transmitted infection. This study retrospectively evaluated the impact of a switch to a real-time PCR assay in the HPV prevalence and genotypes distribution by a quasi-experimental before-and-after approach. Materials and Methods: In total, 1742 samples collected from 1433 patients were analyzed at the UOC Microbiology and Virology of Policlinico of Bari, Italy. HPV DNA detection was performed using initially nested PCR and subsequently multiplex real-time PCR assay. Results: Statistically significant difference in HPV overall prevalence after the introduction of the real-time assay was not detected (48.97% vs. 50.62%). According to different extraction-DNA amplification methods, differences were observed in the prevalence rates of HPV-45, 68, 40, 42, and 43. The lowest prevalence for HPV-45 was observed in the Magna Pure-Real Time PCR group, while HPV-68, 40, 42, and 43 were less observed in the Qiagen-Real Time PCR group. After, a multivariate logistic regression, an increase in the prevalence of HPV-42 (aOR: 4.08, 95% CI: 1.71–9.73) was associated with the multiplex real-time PCR assay. Conclusions: Although this study is a not a direct comparison between two diagnostic methods because it has a sequential structure, it serves to verify the impact of a new molecular assay on HPV distribution. Moreover, the stability of HPV prevalence over time suggests that the population composition and the behavioral variables did not likely change during the observation period. Our study proposes that the introduction of a molecular test for HPV detection may be related to changes of HPV genotypes distribution.

Keywords: HPV; sexually transmitted diseases (STDs); laboratory methods; PCR; genotypes; surveillance; epidemiology

---

1. Introduction

Human papillomavirus (HPV) is still the most prevalent viral sexually-transmitted infection either in men or women. Clinically, it is characterized by a wide spectrum of manifestations, including premalignant lesions that regress spontaneously and malignant lesions evolving to cervical cancer (CC) [1].

Worldwide, although cervical screening programs have contributed to a decrease in the incidence, CC continues to be the second most common cancer among women, with an estimated 266,000 deaths for year [2].

Nevertheless, the use of combined tests to detect the presence of HPV DNA together with conventional cytology examination has been shown to greatly improve the ability to detect the pre-cancerous states [3,4]. Nowadays, with the aim of detecting HPV DNA a wide variety of laboratory diagnostic methods characterized by different grade of sensitivity and specificity are developed [5–8].

Until a few years ago, PCR followed by the nucleic acid hybridization techniques were used to detect HPV genotypes. When compared to conventional cytology, these techniques provided more detailed information regarding HPV genotypes [9].

Afterwards, for HPV diagnosis real-time PCR techniques were introduced. Their performance has significantly improved both the hands-on time and decreased contamination rates.

This study covers three years of routine diagnostic data on HPV DNA and aims to retrospectively evaluate the impact on HPV prevalence and HPV genotypes distribution of a switch from a nested-based PCR to a real-time based PCR on genital samples collected from patients in the Apulia region. To address this issue, a quasi-experimental approach for evaluating the effect of the real-time based PCR on the HPV prevalence and the prevalence of the single viral genotypes was based on the application of multiple logistic regression.

2. Materials and Methods

2.1. Clinical HPV Isolates and Patient Population Characteristics

From January 2012 to December 2014, 1742 consecutive samples, including 1605 cervico-vaginal swabs from 1328 females and 137 urethral swabs from 105 males were collected. Multi samples for some patients were due to retesting in different times.

Specimens were transferred to the laboratory of Molecular Biology, U.O.C. Microbiology and Virology, Azienda Ospedaliera-Universitaria, Policlinico of Bari, where they were analyzed.

All procedures performed in studies involving human participants were in accordance with the ethical standards.

Sample information (date of sampling, ward, type of specimen, testing results) together with the data of patients for whom molecular testing was performed (i.e., age and sex) were recorded in an anonymous database by changing sensitive data into alphanumeric codes. No clinical data associated with these specimens were available.

All procedures performed in studies involving human participants were in accordance with the ethical standards of the institutional and/or national research committee and with the 1964 Helsinki declaration and its later amendments or comparable ethical standards. For this type of study, formal consent is not required. This study was approved by Ethics Committee (No. 5481, 13 December 2017) Azienda Ospedaliero-Universitaria "Consorziale Policlinico," Bari.

2.2. Treatment of Samples

A total of 2 mL of phosphate-buffered saline (pH 7.4) (Sigma-Aldrich, Milano, Italy) was added to cervical-vaginal swabs, collected by a rigid cotton-tipped swab applicator (Nuova Aptaca, Cannelli, Italy), and vortexed. Then, 1 mL of phosphate buffered saline (Sigma, Milano, Italy) was added to urethral swabs and vortexed. Finally, all samples were transferred to microcentrifuge tubes and they were stored at −20 °C until processing. To extract viral nucleic acids, microcentrifuge tubes were centrifuged at rcf = 15,700× *g* for 15 min at 7 °C. The majority of supernatant was discarded but 200 μL of supernatant was retained to resuspend the pellet.

2.3. DNA Isolation (QIAcube System vs. MagNa Pure 96 System)

From January 2012 to December 2013, DNA extraction was performed by automated QIAcube System (Qiagen, Hilden, Germany), following the manufacturer's protocols.

From January 2014 to December 2014, the vilrral nucleic acids were extracted from the resuspended pellet using the automated MagNa Pure 96 system (Roche Diagnostics GmbH, Mennheim, Germany) according to the manufacturer's instructions.

2.4. DNA Amplification (Nested-PCR vs. Multiplex Real-Time PCR)

From January 2012 to June 2013, the extracted DNA samples were subject to a nested polymerase chain reaction (PCR) amplification, using Ampliquality HPV-HS Bio Kit (AB Analitica, Padova, Italy) following the manufacturer's instructions.

The method provides for a first amplification of the viral genome L1 region, followed by a nested PCR with biotinylated primers. PCR products were analyzed using 3% agarose gel electrophoresis with ethidium bromide to display DNA under ultraviolet light. Subsequently, PCR products were typed by using Reverse Line Blot Hybridization Ampliquality HPV-Type Kit (AB Analitica, Padova, Italy).

To assess the suitability of extracted DNA, the thiosulfate sulfurtransferase (TST) gene region (202 bp) was amplified at the first amplification.

From July 2013 to December 2014, the extracted DNA samples were subject to multiplex real-time PCR (mRT-PCR) by Anyplex^{TM} II HPV 28 Detection System (Seegene, Seoul, Korea), which targets the viral L1 region and provides simultaneous detection and genotyping of 28 HPV-types. Briefly, the detection consists of two PCR reactions (panel A and B). The panel A includes 14 high-risk HPV (HR/HPV)-types, while the panel B includes 5 HR and 9 low-risk (LR)-types. PCR was performed on the CFX96 Real-Time PCR system (Bio-Rad, Hercules, CA, USA).

2.5. Statistical Analysis

Differences in HPV prevalence were evaluated by Chi-Squared test and Fisher's test as appropriate. *p*-values were corrected by Benjamini and Hochberg's (BH) procedure with False Discovery Rate (FDR) <1% [10]. Pairwise comparison was performed on each statistically significant combination group of extraction and amplification methods by Fisher's test and BH's correction with FDR <1%.

To assess the association of the real-time assay on the prevalence of the HPV overall infection and the prevalence of each HPV genotype (dependent variables) on the analyzed samples (samples dataset), logistic regression analysis was performed. Due to the lack of birth date for 102 patients, missing ages were imputed by multiple imputation by fully conditional specification implemented in the Multivariate Imputation by Chained Equations (MICE) package implemented in the environment R. A predictive mean matching imputation model was specified on the assumption of missing at random ages and the number of iterations was set to 20. In particular, 50 imputed data sets were generated. For each dataset, a logistic regression model was generated, and the 50 models were pooled together by the function pool of the package mice. Globally, 27 logistic regression models were evaluated. All *p*-values collected from the logistic regression models were corrected for multiple comparisons by BH procedure with FDR < 1%.

Logistic regression analysis is based on the assumption of independence of the variables. To verify this assumption, a reduced dataset only containing the first sample for each patient (patient dataset) was generated and all analyses were repeated on it. Odds ratio estimations of the logistic regression models based on the samples and the patients' datasets were compared.

Calculations of all statistical tests were performed by the open source environment R [11].

3. Results

From 1 January 2012 to 31 December 2014, 1742 samples (1605 cervical-vaginal and 137 urethral swabs) from 1433 patients (1328 female and 105 male patients, Female to Male ratio = 12.64) were analyzed.

During the observation period, the number of analyzed samples increased with time from a minimum value of 306 in 2012 to an intermediate value of 666 and to a maximum value of 770 in 2014. Moreover, after the introduction of the real-time assay an increase of analyzed cervico-vaginal swabs (87.66% vs. 94.12%) and a percentage decrease of urethral swabs (12.34% vs. 5.88%) was observed.

From January 2012 to the end of June 2013, 535 samples were extracted by QIAcube System (Qiagen, Hilden, Germany) followed by a nested-PCR technique. From July 2013 to the end of December 2013, 437 specimens were extracted by QIAcube followed by mRT-PCR. From January to December 2014, 770 samples were extracted by MagNa Pure 96 system (Roche) and amplified by mRT-PCR. The HPV prevalence in the three groups was 48.97% (262), 49.65% (217), and 51.16% (394), respectively (Chi-Squared test p-value = 0.719).

After stratification for the three extraction-amplification combinations, significant differences in HPV types prevalence rates were observed for HPV-45, 68, 40, 42, and 43. In particular, the lowest prevalence for HPV-45 was observed in the Magna Pure-Real Time PCR group (0.00%) while HPV-68, 40, 42, and 43 were less observed in the Qiagen-Real Time PCR group (0.37%, 0.00%, 2.06%, and 0.00%, respectively) (Table 1).

Table 1. Human papillomavirus (HPV) genotype prevalence in the three different combination groups of extraction and amplification methods.

HPV Genotype	QIAcube-Nested PCR *n*, (%)	QIAcube-Real Time PCR *n*, (%)	Magna Pure-Real Time PCR *n*, (%)	*p*-Value	BH-Correction
HPV-16	64 (8.31%)	55 (10.28%)	47 (10.76%)	0.29	NS
HPV-18	21 (2.73%)	10 (1.87%)	9 (2.06%)	0.58	NS
HPV-31	68 (8.83%)	36 (6.73%)	25 (5.72%)	0.11	NS
HPV-33	16 (2.08%)	10 (1.87%)	7 (1.60%)	0.85	NS
HPV-35	10 (1.30%)	7 (1.31%)	6 (1.37%)	1.00	NS
HPV-39	20 (2.60%)	6 (1.12%)	11 (2.52%)	0.14	NS
HPV-45	10 (1.30%)	16 (2.99%)	0 (0.00%)	<0.01	S
HPV-51	30 (3.90%)	7 (1.31%)	17 (3.89%)	0.01	NS
HPV-52	19 (2.47%)	10 (1.87%)	10 (2.29%)	0.80	NS
HPV-53	70 (9.09%)	26 (4.86%)	34 (7.78%)	0.01	NS
HPV-56	31 (4.03%)	14 (2.62%)	13 (2.97%)	0.36	NS
HPV-58	30 (3.90%)	24 (4.49%)	15 (3.43%)	0.72	NS
HPV-59	21 (2.73%)	8 (1.50%)	11 (2.52%)	0.33	NS
HPV-66	30 (5.32%)	2 (3.18%)	14 (4.81%)	0.17	NS
HPV-68	30 (3.90%)	2 (0.37%)	14 (3.20%)	<0.01	S
HPV-73	22 (82.86%)	20 (3.74%)	15 (3.43%)	0.66	NS
HPV-82	3 (0.39%)	3 (0.56%)	3 (0.69%)	0.76	NS
HPV-6	46 85.97%)	25 (4.67%)	16 (3.66%)	0.20	NS
HPV-11	18 (2.34%)	7 (1.31%)	2 (0.46%)	0.03	NS
HPV-40	16 (2.08%)	0 (0.00%)	8 (1.83%)	<0.01	S
HPV-42	102 (13.25%)	11 (2.06%)	46 (10.53%)	<0.01	S
HPV-43	14 (1.82%)	0 (0.00%)	4 (0.92%)	<0.01	S
HPV-44	19 (2.47%)	3 (0.56%)	10 (2.29%)	0.02	NS
HPV-54	52 6.75	29 (5.42%)	25 (5.72%)	0.60	NS
HPV-61	27 3.51	12 (2.24%)	23 (5.26%)	0.04	NS
HPV-70	12 1.56	11 (2.06%)	6 (1.37%)	0.70	NS

NS: Non-Significant; S: Significant. p-values were calculated on a 2×3 matrix by Fisher's test and then corrected by Benjamini and Hochberg's correction (False Discovery Rate (FDR) <1%).

In particular, after pairwise comparison, QIAcube-real time combination resulted in higher HPV-45 prevalence compared to Magna Pure-Real Time PCR (2.99% vs. 0.00%), in lower HPV-68, HPV-40, HPV-42 prevalence rates compared to both Magna Pure-Real Time PCR and QIAcube-Nested PCR (HPV-68: 0.37% vs. 3.20% and 0.37% vs. 3.90%, respectively; HPV-40: 0.00% vs. 1.83% and 0.00% vs. 2.08%, respectively; HPV-42: 2.06% vs. 10.53% and 2.06% vs. 13.25%, respectively) and in lower HPV-40 prevalence compared to QIAcube-Nested PCR (0.00% vs. 1.82%).

On logistic regression analysis, the introduction of real-time assay was associated with an increase of HPV-42 (aOR: 4.08, 95% CI: 1.71–9.73) (Table 2). Moreover, the logistic regression analysis did not reveal the presence of background trends. The comparison of the estimates of the odds ratios of the models built on the samples dataset and the patients dataset revealed absolute differences <1 in the majority of cases (Table 2).

Table 2. Evaluation by logistic regression models of introduction of real time assay on HPV and HPV genotypes detection.

Dependent Variable	Samples Dataset Odds Ratio (95% Confidence Interval)					Patients Datase tOdds Ratio (95% Confidence Interval)				
	Age	Sex (M vs. F)	Year	DNA Extraction	Test Type	Age	Sex (M vs. F)	Year	DNA Extraction	Test Type
HPV-16 →	0.99 (0.97–1.01)	0.69 (0.34–1.4)	1.35 (0.75–2.44)	1.81 (0.88–3.71)	0.84 (0.51–1.39)	0.98 (0.96–1)	0.86 (0.4–1.84)	1.11 (0.56–2.18)	1.44 (0.64–3.23)	1.05 (0.58–1.89)
HPV-18 →	0.98 (0.94–1.01)	0.7 (0.16–2.97)	0.7 (0.19–2.55)	0.55 (0.12–2.5)	1.12 (0.34–3.67)	0.97 (0.94–1.01)	0.85 (0.2–3.65)	0.93 (0.24–3.56)	0.74 (0.15–3.59)	1.02 (0.31–3.39)
HPV-31 →	**0.95 (0.93–0.97)**	0.7 (0.32–1.57)	1.65 (0.8–3.41)	1.1 (0.46–2.63)	0.55 (0.3–1)	**0.96 (0.94–0.98)**	0.74 (0.29–1.89)	1.56 (0.69–3.53)	0.87 (0.33–2.33)	0.54 (0.27–1.1)
HPV-33 →	0.97 (0.93–1.01)	0.39 (0.05–2.91)	2.14 (0.52–8.76)	1.77 (0.33–9.45)	0.56 (0.18–1.69)	0.97 (0.93–1.01)	0.5 (0.07–3.77)	2 (0.46–8.61)	1.96 (0.34–11.26)	0.61 (0.19–1.97)
HPV-35 →	0.97 (0.92–1.01)	0 (0–Inf)	2.68 (0.51–14.14)	3.27 (0.46–23.19)	0.56 (0.17–1.86)	0.97 (0.92–1.02)	0 (0–Inf)	1.83 (0.29–11.32)	1.65 (0.18–14.89)	0.57 (0.12–2.57)
HPV-39 →	**0.92 (0.89–0.96)**	0.37 (0.05–2.74)	0.22 (0.02–1.96)	0.23 (0.02–2.39)	5.24 (0.67–41.05)	**0.89 (0.84–0.94)**	0.45 (0.06–3.46)	0.2 (0.02–1.88)	0.25 (0.02–2.64)	4.5 (0.57–35.81)
HPV-45 →	1.01 (0.97–1.05)	1.71 (0.48–6.04)	1.74 (0.6–5.04)	0 (0–Inf)	0 (0–Inf)	1.01 (0.96–1.06)	2 (0.42–9.44)	1.06 (0.27–4.1)	0 (0–Inf)	0 (0–Inf)
HPV-51 →	**0.94 (0.91–0.98)**	0.25 (0.03–1.82)	0.95 (0.19–4.82)	0.99 (0.18–5.57)	2.73 (0.79–9.48)	0.95 (0.92–0.99)	0.33 (0.04–2.48)	1.1 (0.22–5.57)	0.92 (0.16–5.32)	2.09 (0.59–7.39)
HPV-52 →	1.01 (0.97–1.04)	0 (0–Inf)	0.82 (0.23–2.97)	0.92 (0.2–4.18)	1.26 (0.39–4.08)	1.01 (0.98–1.04)	0 (0–Inf)	0.98 (0.27–3.59)	0.92 (0.2–4.32)	0.99 (0.3–3.26)
HPV-53 →	0.98 (0.96–1)	0.82 (0.37–1.82)	0.6 (0.25–1.47)	0.53 (0.2–1.43)	2.22 (1.01–4.9)	0.98 (0.96–1)	0.83 (0.33–2.13)	0.69 (0.27–1.82)	0.61 (0.21–1.78)	1.89 (0.81–4.43)
HPV-56 →	0.99 (0.97–1.02)	0.84 (0.26–2.77)	0.64 (0.18–2.22)	0.49 (0.12–2)	1.67 (0.54–5.21)	1 (0.97–1.03)	1.13 (0.34–3.76)	0.64 (0.16–2.64)	0.49 (0.1–2.36)	2.06 (0.58–7.34)
HPV-58 →	1 (0.97–1.02)	0.17 (0.02–1.27)	1.91 (0.8–4.53)	1.68 (0.58–4.91)	0.52 (0.24–1.09)	1 (0.97–1.02)	0.24 (0.03–1.78)	1.74 (0.66–4.57)	1.52 (0.46–4.98)	0.56 (0.24–1.31)
HPV-59 →	0.98 (0.94–1.01)	0.78 (0.18–3.31)	0.42 (0.08–2.19)	0.36 (0.06–2.25)	2.51 (0.54–11.61)	0.99 (0.95–1.02)	0.51 (0.07–3.81)	0.25 (0.03–2.18)	0.24 (0.02–2.41)	4.58 (0.58–36.14)
HPV-66 →	0.97 (0.94–0.99)	0.54 (0.17–1.76)	1.04 (0.36–3.04)	0.91 (0.27–3.04)	1.41 (0.59–3.4)	0.97 (0.95–1)	0.47 (0.11–1.97)	1.03 (0.34–3.16)	1.01 (0.28–3.57)	1.43 (0.56–3.66)
HPV-68 →	1 (0.97–1.03)	0 (0–Inf)	0 (0–Inf)	0 (0–Inf)	26,437,379.16 (0–Inf)	0.98 (0.95–1.02)	0 (0–Inf)	0 (0–Inf)	0 (0–Inf)	27,473,819.35 (0–Inf)
HPV-73 →	0.97 (0.94–1)	0.9 (0.32–2.58)	1.16 (0.46–2.94)	1.35 (0.42–4.28)	0.68 (0.3–1.57)	0.98 (0.95–1.01)	1.08 (0.37–3.12)	1.33 (0.52–3.39)	1.63 (0.49–5.41)	0.58 (0.25–1.37)
HPV-82 →	0.95 (0.87–1.03)	1.6 (0.19–13.52)	0.93 (0.06–15.13)	1.59 (0.06–40)	1.5 (0.15–14.6)	0.95 (0.88–1.03)	1.83 (0.21–15.6)	1.03 (0.06–16.92)	1.54 (0.06–38.94)	1.44 (0.15–14.1)
HPV-6 →	0.98 (0.96–1.01)	2.39 (1.24–4.61)	1.36 (0.58–3.19)	0.78 (0.27–2.19)	0.63 (0.3–1.34)	0.99 (0.96–1.01)	2.23 (1.01–4.93)	1.19 (0.43–3.27)	0.81 (0.25–2.65)	0.98 (0.41–2.34)
HPV-11 →	1 (0.96–1.04)	**10.21 (4.2–24.82)**	1.83 (0.32–10.34)	0.26 (0.03–2.61)	0.29 (0.05–1.61)	1 (0.94–1.05)	**11.4 (3.41–38.09)**	1.01 (0.14–7.47)	0.12 (0.01–2.22)	0.3 (0.03–3.37)
HPV-40 →	0.99 (0.94–1.03)	1.5 (0.34–6.6)	0.93 (0–Inf)	0.83 (0–Inf)	16,082,537.86 (0–Inf)	0.98 (0.93–1.03)	1.04 (0.13–8.11)	0.91 (0–Inf)	1.1 (0–Inf)	18,565,563.58 (0–Inf)
HPV-42 →	**0.97 (0.96–0.99)**	0.36 (0.13–1.01)	1.28 (0.38–4.29)	1.08 (0.3–3.81)	**4.08 (1.71–9.73)**	0.97 (0.95–0.99)	0.38 (0.12–1.23)	1.2 (0.34–4.25)	1.15 (0.3–4.31)	**4.31 (1.67–11.1)**
HPV-43 →	0.98 (0.94–1.03)	2.23 (0.49–10.05)	0.9 (0–Inf)	0.41 (0–Inf)	21,853,475.78 (0–Inf)	0.99 (0.94–1.04)	2.87 (0.62–13.23)	0.87 (0–Inf)	0.34 (0–Inf)	9,855,453.89 (0–Inf)
HPV-44 →	1.02 (0.99–1.06)	1.03 (0.24–4.45)	0.61 (0.05–6.85)	0.54 (0.04–6.84)	5.44 (0.69–42.88)	1.02 (0.98–1.06)	1.73 (0.39–7.69)	0.7 (0.06–7.9)	0.5 (0.04–6.72)	3.45 (0.42–28.42)
HPV-54 →	0.98 (0.96–1)	0.61 (0.24–1.55)	1.76 (0.8–3.86)	1.48 (0.59–3.76)	0.72 (0.38–1.36)	0.98 (0.95–1)	0.4 (0.1–1.67)	1.08 (0.4–2.89)	1.18 (0.38–3.68)	1.17 (0.51–2.71)
HPV-61 →	1.02 (0.99–1.04)	0.44 (0.1–1.82)	1.51 (0.45–5.06)	2.37 (0.62–9.04)	2.05 (0.82–5.12)	1 (0.97–1.03)	0.32 (0.04–2.39)	2.34 (0.55–10.06)	3.11 (0.63–15.39)	1.54 (0.56–4.26)
HPV-70 →	1.04 (1–1.07)	1.52 (0.44–5.2)	2.23 (0.64–7.83)	1.82 (0.37–9.04)	0.46 (0.15–1.4)	1.05 (1.01–1.09)	2.25 (0.49–10.4)	1.03 (0.17–6.41)	0.64 (0.07–5.73)	1.01 (0.18–5.6)
HPV →	**0.98 (0.97–0.99)**	0.83 (0.57–1.22)	1.24 (0.86–1.79)	1.17 (0.75–1.81)	0.84 (0.6–1.16)	0.98 (0.97–0.99)	0.84 (0.54–1.31)	**1.11 (0.74–1.66)**	1.08 (0.67–1.75)	0.92 (0.64–1.33)

Bolded: Statistically significant after BH's correction. Each variable in the first column was the dependent variable (Absence vs. Presence) of the model while the independent variables were the Age (linear variable), the Sex (Male vs. Female), the Year of testing (linear variable), the DNA Extraction method (Qiagen vs. Magna Pure) and the Test Type (Real-Time PCR assay vs. Nested assay). Each regression analysis was performed on both the samples and the patient datasets.

4. Discussion

This study evaluated the HPV positivity rates and the HPV genotypes distribution before and after the switch from a nested-based PCR to a real-time PCR on a three-year observation window. Multivariate analysis showed that the HPV prevalence was not affected by the introduction of the new real-time assay. The sensitivity of a nested PCR compared to a real-time amplification method was analyzed by several authors, but the conclusions were not unique [12–14].

On the other hand, some differences in the distribution of HPV genotypes were detected. In particular, the pairwise comparison showed some statistically significant differences in the distribution of HPV-45, 68, 40, 42, and 43. The analysis also highlighted that these differences were due to the QIAcube-Real Time PCR group. Logistic regression analysis only confirmed that the Real Time introduction was associated with an increase of the prevalence of HPV-42 (aOR: 4.08, 95%CI: 1.71–9.73).

Currently, more than 100 distinct molecular tests are available on the global market for the detection of HPV DNA [15]. However, despite the approving of several tests for clinical use in USA and Europe, some tests detect a pool of 12 HPV genotypes (HPV 16, 18, 31, 33, 35, 39, 45, 51, 52, 56, 58, and 59) while other tests also include HPV 66 and 68 [15]. On the other hand, some commercially available tests allow specific HPV genotyping [16]. Some studies reported that genotyping techniques might be useful to improve the triage and follow up of HPV infected women [17]. In fact, some authors suggested that the genotypes 16/18 are related to a more elevated progressive risk [18,19].

An important source of variations is that the detection of specific HPV genotypes may be affected by the different sensitivities of the currently available genotyping methods.

In a study of Del Pino et al. [16] several genotyping tests (Anyplex™ II HPV 28 Detection System, Linear Array HPV genotyping test, Gp5+/6+ PCR-EIA-RH, CLART HPV2 Assay) were compared with Hybrid Capture 2 and a concordance about 80% or higher was reported. In particular, the comparison of the genotype distribution between Anyplex™ and Linear Array, Gp5+/6+ and CLART2, respectively, showed completely different genotypes in five (4.0%), two (2.3%), and three (2.9%) samples.

In a study of Lim et al. [20], Anyplex™ was compared with MolecuTech REBA HPV-ID and HPV DNAChip and the percentage of HPV genotype agreement ranged from 93.7% to 100.0%. However, relatively high rates of discordance between the three assays were reported for HPV 31, 42, and 44. The authors also examined the performance of the assays in the detection of five common HPV genotypes (HPV 16, 18, 45, 52, and 58) and reported that the sensitivity rates varied according to the detection method. In particular, MolecuTech showed a low sensitivity for HPV 52 (42.9%) while Anyplex™ and HPV DNAChip had low sensitivities for HPV 45 (25.0%).

Comparison of Anyplex™ with Euroarray on 150 samples by Latsuzbaia et al. [21] showed a Kappa concordance below 0.7 for HPV 40, 68, 73, and above 0.95 for HPV 11, 16, 18, 33, and 59. Interestingly, a statistically significant difference between assays was detected for HPV 42 genotype since it was more frequently detected by Anyplex™ assay.

Marcuccilli et al. [22] reported that Anyplex™, compared with HPV Sign Genotyping Test, detected more high risk and low risk genotypes. In particular, better agreements were reported for HPV 16, 18, 35, and 70. Statistically significant differences were reported for HPV 31, 51, 52, 53, 56, 58, 59, 66, 73, 6, 42, 44, 54, and 61. These genotypes, except HPV 73, were more frequently detected by Anyplex™ assay.

Differences in HPV genotype detection were also reported by Estrade et al. [23] after comparison of Anyplex™ with PGMY-CHUV assay. In particular, HPV 40, 42, 54, and 68 were significantly more frequently detected by AnyplexTM. On the contrary, HPV 51 was more frequently detected by the PGMY-CHUV assay.

The sequential design does not permit to infer the different sensitivities or specificities of the two diagnostic tests. However, the quasi-experimental approach of the study may be advantageous to acquire some preliminary information to better design subsequent studies or to speculate regarding the clinical usefulness of a new diagnostic assay in a relatively cheap manner. In particular, the latter option may be of some interest in a lack of funds context. To our knowledge, this is the first time that a quasi-experimental before-and-after approach has been applied to the evaluation of a new assay for the HPV evaluation. In particular, the data suggest that the introduction of Real-Time PCR did not affect the HPV prevalence, but it was associated with modification of the distribution of HPV-42. Other studies will be needed to clarify the reasons for these variations. However, other limits of this study must be considered. In particular, the temporal window is quite short and the influence of pluriannual trends cannot be excluded. Moreover, the composition of the population analyzed is not known and the differences in the distribution of the HPV genotypes may reflect differences in the behaviors or risk factors of the analyzed patients. However, the presence of background trends was also excluded by the logistic regression analysis and this makes it possible to assume that the behavioral and social parameters of the analyzed population have not changed over time.

Despite these limits, such study suggests to carefully evaluate the introduction of a new type test for HPV also regarding the impact on the distribution of HPV genotypes. In particular, it may be considered as a potential confounding factor for evaluation of public health programs to control HPV spreading in the populations. At the same time, our study highlights the importance to carefully evaluate temporal dynamics with multivariate methods. Related to this, the accumulation of more rich surveillance data should be encouraged to ensure that demographic shifts in infection patterns could be accurately monitored.

5. Conclusions

Having in mind that any technical innovation is usually related to new perspectives for both clinical and technical development over time, the results obtained suggest that the temporal distribution of HPV genotypes might be influenced by the diagnostic methods that are performed.

This study is not a direct comparison of two diagnostic methods because it has a sequential design. In summary, with univariate analysis significant differences were observed in the prevalence rates of HPV-45, 68, 40, 42, and 43. The lowest prevalence for HPV-45 was observed in the Magna Pure-Real Time PCR group, while HPV-68, 40, 42, and 43 were less observed in the Qiagen-Real Time PCR group.

With logistic regression analysis, the introduction of the real-time assay was associated with an increase in HPV-42. Furthermore, the logistic regression analysis did not reveal the presence of underlying trends. It is possible that the difference in the HPV-42 distribution detected after the switch to the real-time test could be related to the different sensitivities of the two diagnostic assays or to the presence of cross-reactions.

An important limitation of this kind of study is the potential confounding effect of some variables (secular trends, changes in population composition, or behavioral risks). Unfortunately, these data were not available for the analysis. However, despite the increase in number of subjects tested, the stability of HPV prevalence over time suggests that the population composition and the behavioral variables did not likely change during the observation period.

Therefore, this parameter should be taken into the consideration when a multivariate statistical model is represented, and further clinical studies could increase knowledge on the prevalence of HPV based on the use of different methods.

Author Contributions: Conceptualization, R.D.P.; Data curation, L.R., A.A. and L.S.; Investigation, R.D.P., L.R., G.A., R.M. and A.A.; Methodology, R.D.P., L.R., G.A., R.M., D.D.C. and L.S.; Project administration, R.D.P. and L.S.; Supervision, R.D.P. and L.S.; Validation, R.D.P., L.R. and D.D.C.; Writing—original draft, A.A.; Writing—review and editing, L.S.

Funding: This study did not receive funding.

Acknowledgments: We are extremely thankful to Christopher Williams, University of Foggia, for the text revision.

Conflicts of Interest: The authors declare no conflict of interest.

References

1. Stanley, M. Pathology and epidemiology of HPV infection in females. *Gynecol. Oncol.* **2010**, *117*, S5–S10. [CrossRef] [PubMed]

2. The Global Cancer Observatory (GCO) Is an Interactive Web-Based Platform Presenting Global Cancer Statistics to Inform Cancer Control and Research. Available online: http://globocan.iarc.fr/Default.aspx (accessed on 5 June 2019).
3. Schiller, J.T.; Lowy, D.R. Prospects for Cervical Cancer Prevention by Human Papillomavirus Vaccination: Table 1. *Cancer Res.* **2006**, *66*, 10229–10232. [CrossRef] [PubMed]
4. Wright, T.C. Jr.; Schiffman, M.; Solomon, D.; Cox, J.T.; Garcia, F.; Goldie, S.; Hatch, K.; Noller, K.L.; Roach, N.; Runowicz, C.; et al. Interim guidance for the use of human papillomavirus DNA testing as an adjunct to cervical cytology for screening. *Obstet. Gynecol.* **2004**, *103*, 304–309. [CrossRef] [PubMed]
5. Albrecht, V.; Chevallier, A.; Magnone, V.; Barbry, P.; Vandenbos, F.; Bongain, A.; Lefebvre, J.C.; Giordanengo, V. Easy and fast detection and genotyping of high-risk human papillomavirus by dedicated DNA microarrays. *J. Virol. Methods* **2006**, *137*, 236–244. [CrossRef] [PubMed]
6. Gheit, T.; Landi, S.; Gemignani, F.; Snijders, P.J.F.; Vaccarella, S.; Franceschi, S.; Canzian, F.; Tommasino, M. Development of a Sensitive and Specific Assay Combining Multiplex PCR and DNA Microarray Primer Extension to Detect High-Risk Mucosal Human Papillomavirus Types. *J. Clin. Microbiol.* **2006**, *44*, 2025–2031. [CrossRef]
7. Oh, Y.; Bae, S.M.; Kim, Y.W.; Choi, H.S.; Nam, G.H.; Han, S.J.; Park, C.H.; Cho, Y.; Han, B.D.; Ahn, W.S. Polymerase chain reaction-based fluorescent Luminex assay to detect the presence of human papillomavirus types. *Cancer Sci.* **2007**, *98*, 549–554. [CrossRef]
8. Sotlar, K.; Diemer, D.; Dethleffs, A.; Hack, Y.; Stubner, A.; Vollmer, N.; Menton, S.; Menton, M.; Dietz, K.; Wallwiener, D.; et al. Detection and Typing of Human Papillomavirus by E6 Nested Multiplex PCR. *J. Clin. Microbiol.* **2004**, *42*, 3176–3184. [CrossRef]
9. Villa, L.L.; Denny, L. CHAPTER 7 Methods for detection of HPV infection and its clinical utility. *Int. J. Gynecol. Obstet.* **2006**, *94*, S71–S80. [CrossRef]
10. Hochberg, Y.; Benjamini, Y. More powerful procedures for multiple significance testing. *Stat. Med.* **1990**, *9*, 811–818. [CrossRef]
11. R Core Team. R: A Language and Environment for Statistical Computing. Available online: https://www.R-project.org/ (accessed on 5 June 2019).
12. Kim, H.S.; Kim, D.M.; Neupane, G.P.; Lee, Y.M.; Yang, N.W.; Jang, S.J.; Jung, S.I.; Park, K.H.; Park, H.R.; Lee, C.S.; et al. Comparison of Conventional, Nested, and Real-Time PCR Assays for Rapid and Accurate Detection of Vibrio vulnificus. *J. Clin. Microbiol.* **2008**, *46*, 2992–2998. [CrossRef]
13. Pasternak, A.O.; Adema, K.W.; Bakker, M.; Jurriaans, S.; Berkhout, B.; Cornelissen, M.; Lukashov, V.V. Highly Sensitive Methods Based on Seminested Real-Time Reverse Transcription-PCR for Quantitation of Human Immunodeficiency Virus Type 1 Unspliced and Multiply Spliced RNA and Proviral DNA. *J. Clin. Microbiol.* **2008**, *46*, 2206–2211. [CrossRef] [PubMed]
14. Kim, D.M.; Park, G.; Kim, H.S.; Lee, J.Y.; Neupane, G.P.; Graves, S.; Stenos, J. Comparison of conventional, nested, and real-time quantitative PCR for diagnosis of scrub typhus. *J. Clin. Microbiol.* **2011**, *49*, 607–612. [CrossRef] [PubMed]
15. Burd, E.M. Human Papillomavirus Laboratory Testing: The Changing Paradigm. *Clin. Microbiol. Rev.* **2016**, *29*, 291–319. [CrossRef] [PubMed]
16. Del Pino, M.; Alonso, I.; Rodriguez-Trujillo, A.; Bernal, S.; Geraets, D.; Guimerà, N. Comparison of the analytical and clinical performance of five tests for the detection of human papillomavirus genital infection. *J. Virol. Methods* **2017**, *248*, 238–243. [CrossRef] [PubMed]
17. Khan, M.J.; Castle, P.E.; Lorincz, A.T.; Wacholder, S.; Sherman, M.; Scott, D.R.; Rush, B.B.; Glass, A.G.; Schiffman, M. The Elevated 10-Year Risk of Cervical Precancer and Cancer in Women with Human Papillomavirus (HPV) Type 16 or 18 and the Possible Utility of Type-Specific HPV Testing in Clinical Practice. *J. Natl. Cancer Inst.* **2005**, *97*, 1072–1079. [CrossRef] [PubMed]
18. Ye, J.; Cheng, B.; Cheng, Y.F.; Yao, Y.L.; Xie, X.; Lu, W.G.; Cheng, X.D. Prognostic value of human papillomavirus 16/18 genotyping in low-grade cervical lesions preceded by mildly abnormal cytology. *J. Zhejiang Univ. Sci. B* **2017**, *18*, 249–255. [CrossRef]
19. Lagos, M.; Van De Wyngard, V.; Poggi, H.; Cook, P.; Viviani, P.; Barriga, M.I.; Pruyas, M.; Ferreccio, C. HPV16/18 genotyping for the triage of HPV positive women in primary cervical cancer screening in Chile. *Infect. Agents Cancer* **2015**, *10*, 916. [CrossRef] [PubMed]

20. Lim, Y.K.; Choi, J.H.; Park, S.; Kweon, O.J.; Park, A.J.; Choi, J. Comparison of Three Different Commercial Kits for the Human Papilloma Virus Genotyping. *J. Clin. Lab. Anal.* **2016**, *30*, 1110–1115. [CrossRef]
21. Latsuzbaia, A.; Tapp, J.; Nguyen, T.; Fischer, M.; Arbyn, M.; Weyers, S.; Mossong, J. Analytical performance evaluation of Anyplex II HPV28 and Euroarray HPV for genotyping of cervical samples. *Diagn. Microbiol. Infect. Dis.* **2016**, *85*, 318–322. [CrossRef]
22. Marcuccilli, F.; Farchi, F.; Mirandola, W.; Ciccozzi, M.; Paba, P.; Bonanno, E.; Perno, C.F.; Ciotti, M. Performance evaluation of Anyplex™II HPV28 detection kit in a routine diagnostic setting:comparison with the HPV Sign® Genotyping Test. *J. Virol. Methods* **2015**, *217*, 8–13. [CrossRef]
23. Estrade, C.; Sahli, R. Comparison of Seegene Anyplex II HPV28 with the PGMY-CHUV assay for human papillomavirus genotyping. *J. Clin. Microbiol.* **2014**, *52*, 607–612. [CrossRef] [PubMed]

medicina

MDPI

Article

Different Patterns of HIV-1 Replication in MACROPHAGES is Led by Co-Receptor Usage

Ana Borrajo [1,2], Alessandro Ranazzi [1], Michela Pollicita [1], Maria Concetta Bellocchi [1], Romina Salpini [1], Maria Vittoria Mauro [3], Francesca Ceccherini-Silberstein [1], Carlo Federico Perno [4], Valentina Svicher [1,*] and Stefano Aquaro [5,*]

1 Department of Experimental Medicine and Surgery, University of Rome Tor Vergata, 00133 Roma, Italy; ana.borrajo@hotmail.com (A.B.); aranazzi@yahoo.com (A.R.); michela.pollicita@uniroma2.it (M.P.); mariac.bellocchi@gmail.com (M.C.B.); rsalpini@yahoo.it (R.S); ceccherini@med.uniroma2.it (F.C.-S.)
2 Group of Virology and Pathogenesis, Galicia Sur Health Research Institute (IIS Galicia Sur)-Complexo Hospitalario Universitario de Vigo, SERGAS-UVigo, 36312 Vigo, Spain
3 Department of Microbiology and Virology, Complex Operative Unit (UOC), Hospital of Cosenza, 87100 Cosenza, Italy; m.v.mauro@virgilio.it
4 Department of Microbiology and Clinic Microbiology, University of Milan, 20162 Milan, Italy; cf.perno@uniroma2.it
5 Department of Pharmacy, Health and Nutritional Sciences, University of Calabria, 87036 Rende, Italy
* Correspondence: valentina.svicher@uniroma2.it (V.S.); aquaro@uniroma2.it (S.A.); Tel.: +39-333-238-1462 (V.S.); +39-392-341-8032 (S.A.)

Received: 21 March 2019; Accepted: 11 June 2019; Published: 21 June 2019

Abstract: *Background and objectives:* To enter the target cell, HIV-1 binds not only CD4 but also a co-receptor β-chemokine receptor 5 (CCR5) or α chemokine receptor 4 (CXCR4). Limited information is available on the impact of co-receptor usage on HIV-1 replication in monocyte-derived macrophages (MDM) and on the homeostasis of this important cellular reservoir. *Materials and Methods:* Replication (measured by p24 production) of the CCR5-tropic 81A strain increased up to 10 days post-infection and then reached a plateau. Conversely, the replication of the CXCR4-tropic NL4.3 strain (after an initial increase up to day 7) underwent a drastic decrease becoming almost undetectable after 10 days post-infection. The ability of CCR5-tropic and CXCR4-tropic strains to induce cell death in MDM was then evaluated. While for CCR5-tropic 81A the rate of apoptosis in MDM was comparable to uninfected MDM, the infection of CXCR4-tropic NL4.3 in MDM was associated with a rate of 14.3% of apoptotic cells at day 6 reaching a peak of 43.5% at day 10 post-infection. *Results:* This suggests that the decrease in CXCR4-tropic strain replication in MDM can be due to their ability to induce cell death in MDM. The increase in apoptosis was paralleled with a 2-fold increase in the phosphorylated form of p38 compared to WT. Furthermore, microarray analysis showed modulation of proapoptotic and cancer-related genes induced by CXCR4-tropic strains starting from 24 h after infection, whereas CCR5 viruses modulated the expression of genes not correlated with apoptotic-pathways. *Conclusions:* In conclusion, CXCR4-tropic strains can induce a remarkable depletion of MDM. Conversely, MDM can represent an important cellular reservoir for CCR5-tropic strains supporting the role of CCR5-usage in HIV-1 pathogenesis and as a pharmacological target to contribute to an HIV-1 cure.

Keywords: α chemokine receptor 4; β-chemokine receptor 5; human immunodeficiency virus; monocyte-derived macrophages

1. Introduction

Combined antiretroviral therapy (cART) does not eradicate HIV-1 [1,2] due to the early establishment of a long-lived viral reservoir [3–6]. This reservoir can include cells of macrophage lineage where, in contrast to CD4+ lymphocytes, HIV is relatively non cytopathic and can replicate extensively in intracellular compartments in a long-lasting manner [7–10]. HIV-1 infected monocyte-derived macrophages (MDM) are fully capable of producing infectious viral particles when cART is discontinued [11–16] and may play a key role in regulating the disease progression [17].

Over the following decades, after the discovery of CD4 as the main virus receptor [18,19], further studies have demonstrated that the chemokines coreceptors CCR5 and CXCR4 play crucial duties in supporting infection of HIV-1 in target cells.

Binding of chemokine receptors CCR5 or CXCR4 is widely thought to be the cause that stimulates the membrane fusion during HIV-replicative life cycle [19,20]. Infection with HIV-1 is generally initiated by macrophages, slowly replicating, non-syncytium-inducing (NSI) variants [20,21] that utilize CCR5 as a coreceptor [22–24]. In 50% of instances, disease evolution is correlated with the development of syncytium-inducing (SI) variants which at least use CXCR4 [25–28].

The tropism of HIV-1 for specific and relevant cell populations in diverse compartments is determined by the coreceptor utilized by HIV-1 Env for the entrance of the viral particles [28]. For infection of MDM cultures, HIV viruses preferentially utilize CCR5 as a coreceptor [22–26], whereas viruses in T-cells use CXCR4 [27]. Dual-tropic viruses can utilize both coreceptors (CCR5/CXCR4) [29,30]. Thus, the coreceptor particularity of primary HIV-1 isolates is commonly utilized to characterize cellular tropism [31].

Previous studies have shown that CCR5 is present on a wide variety of cells that can be infected by HIV-viruses, including T cells, monocytes and macrophages. A lot of research has shown the existence of CCR5-tropic viruses, which were proficient in replication of primary CD4+ T cells but which could not effectively infect MDM [32–38]. Also, some CCR5-tropic primary HIV-1 strains utilize CXCR4 for input into MDM [32,38]. Hence, the viral determinants that regulate HIV-1 tropism for macrophages are considerably more complicated than the coreceptor specificity of the virus. HIV-1 viruses use CCR5 for their infection, although their primary targets are T cells not macrophages. It is widely agreed that these CCR5 and CXCR4 viruses can replicate in both macrophages as well as in T cells. However, their replication effectiveness changes in different cell classes which depend upon the cellular environment [37,38]. Moreover, viral progeny from macrophages and T cells may have divergent groups of host protein integrated in their viral particle [39].

HIV-mediated patterns of replication in latently infected cells (virus reservoir) have not been completely understood. HIV infections lead to increased expression of specific proteins like B-cell lymphoma 2 (BCL-2), B-cell lymphoma-extra large (BCL-XL), cellular FLICE (FADD-like IL-1β-converting enzyme)-inhibitory protein (cFLIP), Induced myeloid leukemia cell differentiation protein (Mcl-1) [40–42] or downregulation of proteins Bcl-2-associated X protein (BAX), Bcl-2-associated death promoter protein (BAD proteins), Fas-associated protein with death domain (FADD) [42–44]. These factors contribute to regulate the transcription of genes correlated with host defense, cellular anti-oxidant molecules like glutathione and thioredoxin, signal transduction, survival, and the cell cycle, including the cyclin-dependent kinase inhibitor 1A (CDKN1A/p21) gene whose maximum extent of mRNA and protein expression parallels active HIV-1 replication in latent cells.

This work aims at defining: (i) the role of CCR5-tropic and CXCR4- tropic strains in MDM; (ii) assessment of different patterns of replication in this cell type by evaluating the extent of DNA degradation, viral production, p38 MAPK activation and survival gene modulation in CXCR4 and the CCR5 infected MDM.

2. Materials and Methods

2.1. Virus

HIV-1 pNL4-3p10-17 and p81Ap10-17 molecular constructs were obtained from B. Chesebro, (National Institute of Allergy and Infectious Diseases, Hamilton, Montana 59840, USA) and contain the whole HIV-1 genome [45]. The HIV-1 p81A p10-17 clone was generated by replacing the pNL4-3p10-17 a 659 bp long sequence of env. This nucleotide sequence belongs to the R5-tropic HIV-1 Ba-L and includes the V1, V2, V3 variable domains, whereas NL4-3 is a CXCR4-tropic strain, 81A replicates in cells of the MDM lineage. These plasmids were transfected in 293T through the FuGENE 6TM (Roche), a lipidic, not liposomial reagent.

HIV-1 clinical isolates #17 (X4), #6 (R5) and #10 (R5/X4) were obtained from patients enrolled from the Katholieke Universiteit Leuven (Rega institute, Leuven, Belgium) and expanded in peripheral blood mononuclear cells (PBMC).

The laboratory-adapted HIV-1 X4 strain IIIB was expanded in H9 cells and obtained from supernatants at day 8 post infection. The laboratory-adapted HIV-1 adapted R5-tropic strain Ba-L was expanded in MDM [46,47].

All the strains were purified from supernatants of the respective cultures after centrifugation at 20,000 rpm for 2 h, filtered through 0.45 μm filter, DNase I treated, and concentrated with a Centricon Plus-20 membrane with a 100,000 molecular weight cut-off (Millipore Corporation, Bedford, Mass.) to remove contaminating cytokines and growth factors which might interfere with signal transduction analysis. Concentrated virus was stored in aliquots at −70 °C until use. Stock virus titers were determined with a colorimetric reverse transcriptase activity assay (Roche Molecular Biochemicals, Indianapolis, USA).

2.2. Drugs

The prototype bicyclam CXCR4 inhibitor and agonist stromal derived factor (SDF-1alpha) AMD3100, (1-1*-[1,4-phenylenebis(methylene)]-bis(1,4,8,11-tetraazacyclotetradecane) octahydrochloride dihydrate]) synthesized at Johnson Matthey [48–50], and the CCR5 inhibitor, N,N-dimethyl-N-[4-[[[2-(4-methylphenyl) -6,7-dihydro-5H-benzocyclohepten-8-yl] carbonil]amino]benzyl] tetrahydro-2H-pyran-4-aminium chloride (TAK779), a nonpeptide compound with a small molecular weight (Mr 531.13), (Takeda Chemical Industries, Ltd., Osaka, Japan) [51,52], were suspended and aliquoted in Phosphate-buffered saline (PBS) solution, and used to 5 μM and 2 and 10 μg/mL, respectively.

2.3. Cells

Human primary MDM were generated and purified as previously described [53–56]. MDM were derived from PBMCs of healthy donors. Briefly, PBMCs were separated by Ficoll-Hypaque gradient centrifugation and seeded in T25 flasks at a number of 50.10^6 cells in 7 mL Roswell Park Memorial Institute (RPMI) medium 1640 supplemented with 20% heat inactivated, mycoplasma- and endotoxin-free fetal bovine serum (FBS), L-glutamine (1 mM), penicillin (100 U/mL), and streptomycin (100 μg/mL), without exogenous cytokines or growth factors, at 37 °C in a humidified atmosphere enriched with 5% CO2. After five days of culture, non-adherent cells were eliminated with caution by consecutive gentle washings with warmed RPMI 1640, leaving a monolayer of adherent cells which were finally incubated in complete medium [57–59].

The MDM obtained showed a purity exceeding 98% as tested by cytofluorimetric analysis. Expression of CXCR4 and CCR5 in all our MDM cultures was assayed by flow cytometric analysis (FCM) (FACScanTM, Becton Dickinson System, San José, CA) by means of CD184 (CXCR4/fusin) R-phycoerythrin (R-PE)-conjugated mouse anti-human monoclonal antibody and CD195 (CCR5) R-phycoerythrin (R-PE)-conjugated mouse anti-human monoclonal antibody both purchased from BD Pharmingen (Becton Dickinson biosciences, USA). Measurements were performed in at least 3 independent experiments. In each experiment, MDM derived from a single healthy donor.

2.4. Drug Treatment, Infection and Virus Detection

Six days after Ficoll-Hypaque, non-adherent cells were removed, and monocytes were further allowed to differentiate in MDM for four days. Their purity exceeded 98%. For exposure to inhibitor AMD3100 and TAK779, at least twenty-four hours before CXCR4 and CCR5 strain infection, MDM culture medium was removed and replaced with fresh media 20% serum. 45–60 min before infection;

where needed, the drug was added to the cell supernatants at appropriate concentrations (0.4–2 µg/mL for TAK779, and 5 µM for AMD3100) and then MDM were reincubated at 37 °C in a humidified atmosphere enriched with 5% CO2.

Virus challenge was performed for at least 4 h to almost a week by exposing MDM to 3000 up to 7500 pg/mL of p24 (corresponding to, respectively, 400 and 1000 tissue cultures infectious doses 50% per ml (TCID50/mL) of the Laboratory-adapted strain HIV-1 Ba-L) of the all strains described above, followed by extensive washing to remove excess virus.

Virus production was assessed by the HIV-1 p24 gag antigen concentration in culture supernatants using a p24 gag antigen detection kit according to the instructions of the manufacturer (Abbott labs, Pomezia, Italy).

2.5. *Western Blotting of Cell Cultures*

Cells were challenged with IIIB, NL4-3, Ba-L and 81A strains of HIV (whole visions) in warmed media 20% serum at indicated times at 37 °C in a humidified atmosphere enriched with 5% CO_2, incubated for the times indicated and then lysed and subjected to immunoblot analysis. Lysis was performed in ice-cold buffer Radio-Immunoprecipitation Assay (RIPA) (50 mM tris hydroxymethyl aminomethane ((Tris)-HCl), pH 7.4; 250 mM NaCl; 50 mM NaF, EDTA 5 mM; 0,15% Triton X-100) containing a protease and phosphatase inhibitor cocktails (1 mM phenylmethylsulfonyl fluoride; 10 µg/mL pepstatin; 10 µg/mL leupeptin and 1 mm sodium vanadate) and incubated for different times at 4 °C. Cell lysates were then clarified by centrifugation at 13,000 rpm for 10 min at 4 °C.

Protein concentrations were determined by a spectrophotometric assay (Pierce). Immunoblot analysis was performed on cell lysates containing 30 µg protein mixed with Laemmli buffer and boiled for 5 min. Samples were subjected to 10% Sodium dodecyl sulfate-polyacrylamide gel electrophoresis (SDS-PAGE) and transferred to nitrocellulose membranes. The membranes were blocked overnight with 5% Bovine serum Albumine (BSA) in TBS-tween.

A 1:1000 dilution of the lysates was used for the detection of activated MAPK/p38 a polyclonal antibody specific for Phospho-p38 (Thr202/Tyr204), and for total p38 (Cell Signaling Technology, Beverly, MA). (Jackson ImmunoResearch Laboratories). Then, membranes were treated with the corresponding horseradish peroxidase (HRP)-conjugated secondary antibody (1:5000 dilution) (Jackson ImmunoResearch Laboratories). The immunoreactive bands were visualized using enhanced chemiluminescence Western blotting system (Immun-Star HRP Chemiluminescent Kit, Hercules, Ca, USA) according to the manufacturer's instructions (Biorad, Hercules, CA, USA).

Blots were stripped (2% SDS, 62.5 mM Tris, 100 mM mercaptoethanol) for 30 min at 56 °C and washed in PBS containing 0.05% Tween 20, before blocking and reprobing with primary antibody. For the quantification of the phosphorylated and total proteins, the bands on the films were first scanned by the Epson software program and then the images were processed through the Scion Image analysis program (Houston, TX, USA) for the IBM PC based on the popular NIH Image on the Macintosh platform.

2.6. *RNA Isolation and Microarray Analysis*

In different experiments, 81A and NL4-3 infected MDM were incubated in parallel at a dose of 2000 pg/mL of viral p24 from 6 to 24 h of infection, then exposed to 4M guanidinium and total RNA was isolated by the guanidinium-phenol procedure. The isolation of polyA mRNA from each total RNA preparation was obtained by OLIGOTEX mRNA Purification System (Qiagen, Hilden, Germany). cDNA probes for microarray experiments were prepared from 0.5 µg of cellular mRNA by CyScribe post-Labelling Kit (Amersham Biosciences). The CyDye labelled cDNA was purificated by QIAquik PCR purification Kit (Qiagen). For dual colour hybridization we combined Cy3 and Cy5 labelled cDNAs in one tube. The solution protected from light was dried by using a rotary evaporator and adding tRNA (40 γ), Calf Thymus DNA (40 γ) and Cot-1 DNA (1 γ). The dry solution was dissolved in nuclease free water, denatured at 95 °C for 5 min and cooled in ice. Hybridization buffer 4X (supplied in the CyScribe Post-labelling Kit) was added with $\frac{1}{2}$ volume of 100% formammide. Hybridization was performed in an humid hybridization chamber (5X SSC) at 42 °C for 14–18 h, following washing with saline-sodium citrate (SSC) and SDS (*w*/*v*) pre-warmed to 37 °C. Fluorescent-array images were collected for both Cy3 and Cy5 by using a ScanArray Express, Microarray Analysis System Version 2.0 (Perkin-Elmer) and image intensity data were extracted and analysed by using QuantArray Pachard Biochips Software. In particular, QuantArray Software provides automated analysis of color microarray images (automatic scanning and quantitation to measure fluorescence signal at each spot on the array) before exporting data to bioinformatics software packages. Triplicate array positions are used for each gene to avoid signal noise. The human Cancer Chip version 4.0 (Takara) slides were used for microarray analysis and all spots were known. In order to evaluate the inhibition or enhancement of genes expression in terms of mRNA production, a comparison of Cy3 and Cy5 signals intensity was applied.

2.7. Flow Cytometry Measurement of Apoptotic Cells

At established time points of infection (see results), MDM were washed and detached from the 25 flasks with gentle scraping as previously described [60]. MDM were precipitated by centrifugation at 1500 rpm for 5 min at 4 °C. All MDM in the culture, both adherent and non-adherent, were considered in the final count for apoptosis analysis by Flow Cytometry measurement (FCM). Supernatants were removed, then aliquoted, and stored at −80 °C for p24 titration. After washing, MDM were kept in 3 mL of cold PBS, 0.02% EDTA in 10 min at 4 °C, then gently scraped and transferred to the respective tubes and precipitated by centrifugation at 1500 rpm for 5 min at 4 °C. Supernatants were removed and the pellet resuspended in 0.5 mL of Trypan-blue solution for cell count and viability check. Cells were washed with 2 mL PBS cold and centrifuged as described above.

The supernatants were completely removed and 2 mL of 70% ice ethanol was added to permeabilize for 40 min at 4 °C. After washing, cells were centrifuged (1600 rpm/5 min/4 °C), again washed and centrifuged as described above and gently resuspended in 1.0 mL hysotonic Propidium Iodide (PI) solution (Sigma) 50 µg/mL, in PBS and RNase 50 µg/mL) in polipropylen tubes. After rotating for 15 min at room temperature, the tubes were placed at 4 °C for 2 h in the dark. Cells were washed with 2 mL PBS cold, centrifuged at 1500 rpm for 5 min at 4 °C, resuspended in 0.4 mL cold PBS and kept in the dark at 4 °C for not more than 20 min before PI fluorescent measurement. The DNA specific fluorocrome Propidium Iodide (PI) recognized apoptotic cells as a distinct hyplopIoid cell population with a reduced staining below the G0/G1 population of normal diploid cells as results of cell shrinkage, nuclear condensation, internucleosomal DNA fragmentation [61]. The PI fluorescence was measured by Flow Cytometry in FL2-H (FACScanTM, Becton Dickinson System, San Josè, CA, USA) and registered on a logarithmic scale. All the tests were performed in duplicate.

2.8. Statistics

Differences were considered statistically significant at $p \leq 0.05$ by means of a Chi Square test of independence based on a 2 × 2 contingency table. Statistical analyses were carried out with SigmaStat 3.0 (Jandel Scientific, San Rafael, CA, USA).

3. Results

3.1. Different Replicative Kinetics of CXCR4- and CCR5-Dependent HIV Strains in MDM

The first step of this study was to evaluate the efficiency of CCR5-, CXR4- tropic HIV-1 strains to replicate in MDM by measuring p24 production (Figure 1). In particular, p24 production was similar up to day 7 post infection for both CCR5- and CXR4-tropic strains. After 7 days post infection, p24 production of the CCR5-tropic 81A virus underwent a sharp increase up to day 10 and then tended to remain stable up to day 14. Conversely, p24 production of the CXCR4-tropic NL4.3 sharply decreased, becoming almost undetectable starting from day 10 (Figure 1). As a control, pre-treatment with AMD3100 completely abrogated the replication of the CXCR4- tropic NL4.3 in MDM.

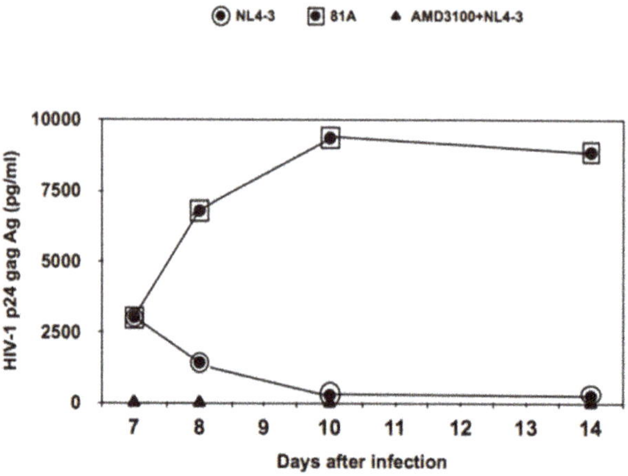

Figure 1. Kinetics of the HIV-1 replication profile in human primary monocyte-derived macrophages (MDM) infected by CXCR4-tropic NL4.3 and or CCR5-tropic 81.A virus. The figure reports p24 production starting from day 7 post-infection. MDM from a healthy donor were infected with a standard dose of p24 gag (3000 pg/mL) of NL4.3 or 81.A. p24 production was measured daily in culture supernatants by a commercially available ELISA (Abbott labs, Pomezia, Italy). Pre-treatment with AMD3100 was performed 1 h before incubation with NL4.3. All tests were performed in triplicate.

3.2. Effect of CXCR4-Tropic NL4.3 and/or CCRR5-Tropic 81.A Dependent HIV Infection Upon DNA Fragmentation

The second step of this study was to investigate the impact of CCR5-tropic 81.A and CXCR4-tropic NL4.3 on inducing apoptosis in MDM by cytofluorometry. In MDM infected with the CXCR4-tropic NL4.3, the percentage of cells in apoptosis progressively increased from day 4 up to day 10 post infection (43.5%) (time point at which the p24 production of the CXCR4-tropic NL4.3 becomes undetectable) and tended to remain stable at around 40% 13 days post infection (Figure 2). As a control, pre-treatment with AMD3100 abrogated the capability of CXCR4-tropic NL4.3 to induce MDM apoptosis (Figure 2). Conversely, very low levels of apoptosis were observed in MDM infected with the CCR5-tropic 81A. Overall findings suggest that the decrease in the replication of the CXCR4-tropic NL4.3 in MDM may be linked to the capability of the viral strain to induce apoptosis of MDM. The capability of CXCR4-tropic strains to favor MDM apoptosis was confirmed in the presence of another laboratory adapted CXCR4-tropic IIIB and in the presence of different CXCR4-tropic clinical isolates. Interestingly, the CCR5/CXCR4-tropic clinical isolate #6 conserved the capability to induce MDM apoptosis despite dual tropism (Figure 3).

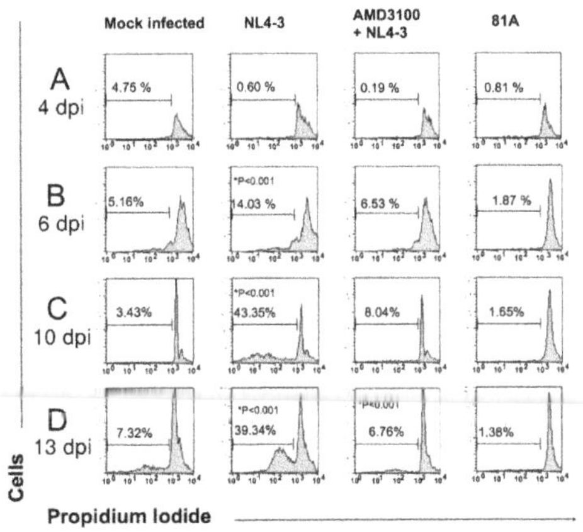

Figure 2. Effects of CXCR4 and CCR5 usage on DNA fragmentation (measure of apoptosis) in MDM. MDM from a healthy donor were infected with 81A (CCR5-tropic strain) or NL4-3 (CXCR4-tropic strain). Percentage of cells undergoing DNA fragmentation was checked: (**A**) 4 days after infection (**B**) 6 days after infection; (**C**) 10 days after infection; (**D**) 13 days after infection. Pretreatment with AMD3100 was performed 1 h before incubation with NL4-3. For HIV infection in MDM, a standard dose of p24 gag (3000 pg/mL) was used. The PI fluorescence was measured by Flow Cytometry in FL2-H (FACScan, Becton Dickinson System, San josè, CA) and registered on a logarithmic scale. The figure is representative of three independent experiments. Differences in NL4-3-infected macrophages are statistically significant ($P < 0.001$, Chi Square test) compared to mock-, 81A-infected and AMD3100-treated macrophages.

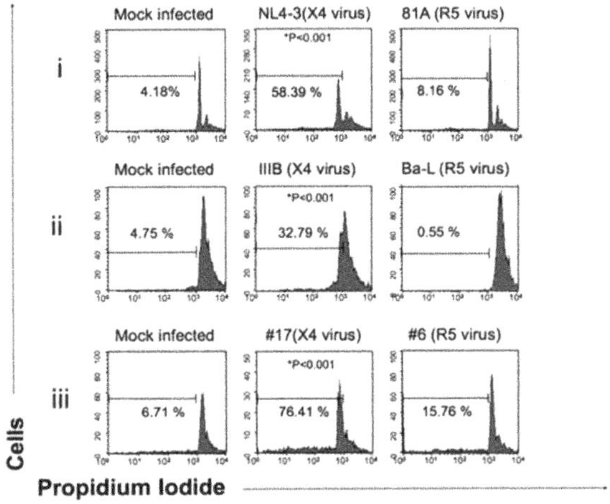

Figure 3. Measure of DNA fragmentation in Human Primary Macrophages infected by X4-tropic virus. The PI fluorescence was measured by Flow Cytometry in FL2-H and registered on a logarithmic scale. All the tests were performed in duplicate. (**i**) NL4-3 and 81A are, respectively, a CXCR4- (X4) and CCR5 (R5)-tropic HIV strains. DNA fragmentation was analyzed to the 10th day of infection (**ii**) IIIB and Ba-L are laboratory-adapted HIV strains using, respectively, X4 and R5 strains. DNA fragmentation was analyzed to the 7th day of infection. (**iii**) #17 and #6 are, respectively, a CXCR4- and CCR5-tropic HIV-1 clinical isolates and DNA fragmentation was analyzed to the 12th day of infection. For the infection, a standard dose of p24 gag (3000 pg/mL) correspondent to 400 TCID50/mL dose of Ba-L was used. * Differences in X4 strain infected macrophages are statistically significative ($P < 0.001$, Chi Squared test) compared to mock infected and R5 strain infected macrophages (see material and methods).

3.3. *Impact of CXCR4-Tropic (CXCR4) and CCR5-Tropic (CCR5) Strains in p38 Activation in MDM*

To further corroborate the capability of CXCR4-tropic strains to favor MDM apoptosis, the detection of the phosphorylated form of the mitogen-activated protein p38/MAPK (phospho- p38) was evaluated. After exposing NL4.3 for 30 min (Figure 4 Lane 9), a 2-fold increase in the detection of the phospho- p38 MAPK was observed compared to MDM exposed to p81A. Thus, NL4-3 induced the activation of the p38/MAPK since early phases of MDM infection (while no effect was observed for 81A) [62]. Similarly, an increase in the detection of the phosphorylated form of p38 was also observed after exposing the CXCR4-tropic IIIB to MDM for 30 min (Figure 5A). Conversely, the detection of the phosphorylated form of p38 was reduced when AMD3100 was used (Figure 5B).

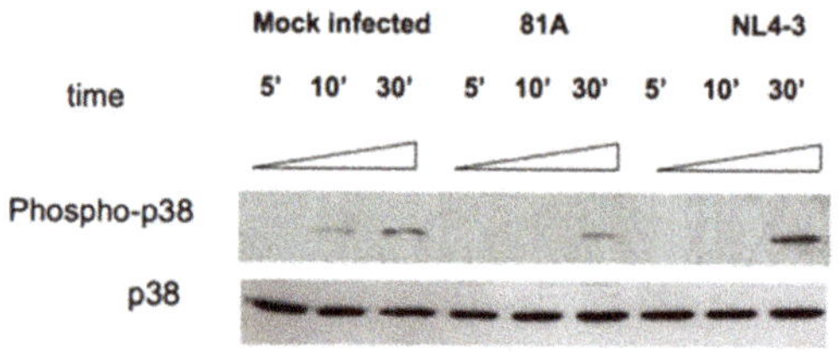

Figure 4. Detection of p38 and phospho p38 by Western Blotting in cell lysates. MDM were infected with 7500 pg/mL of NL4.3 or 81.A. Blots are representative of three experiments using MDM from different donors after exposing NL4.3 and 81.A in MDM for 5, 10 and 30 min.

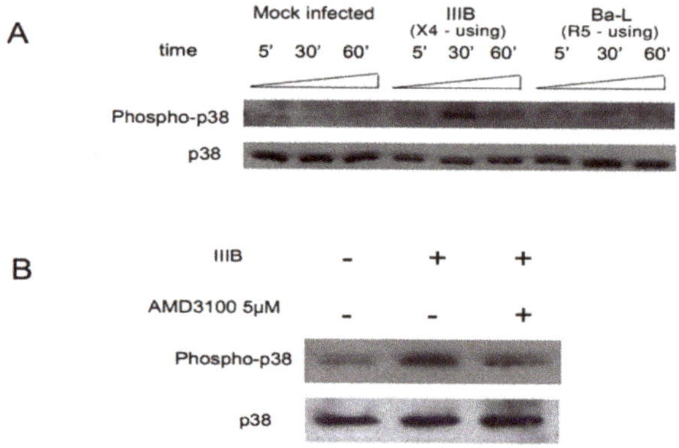

Figure 5. Detection of p38 and phospho p38 by Western Blotting. MDM were infected with 7500 pg/mL of the CXCR4-tropic IIIB and the CCR5-tropic 81.A. (**A**) Cell lysates were subjected to immunoblot analysis with antibodies specific for the total or phosphorylated forms of p38 MAPK (phospho-p38 MAPK [T180/Y182] antibody). (**B**) MDM from HIV-1 negative donor were pretreated for 30 min with (+) or without (−) AMD3100 (5μg/mL) before incubation with IIIB. Blots are representative of three experiments using MDM from different donors.

3.4. *Modulation of Expression of Genes Correlated with Apoptotic Pathways, in a Time-Dependent Manner, by CXCR4-Tropic Strains*

As a final step of this study, we analyzed variation in the transcriptome profile observed in MDM infected by CCR5-tropic or CXCR4-tropic strains. We found that NL4-3, but not 81A, up-regulated many genes in human MDM, including TNF2, Fas (TNFRSF6)-associated via death domain [63], caspase-7, Cytocrome C, KGF [64] and GSPT1/eRF3 [65] but down-regulates survival and cancer genes. These findings indicate that CXCR4-mediated the entry in MDM can up regulate apoptosis-related genes and simultaneously down modulate survival-related genes as Defender against cell death 1(DAD-1) and Cullin 2 (hCUL2), involved in MDM survival after HIV-1 infection. Interestingly, we also observed enhancement in gene activation of pro-inflammatory Matrix metalloproteinase 9 (MMP9 gelatinase B, 92kD gelatinase, 92kD type IV collagenase) by the CXCR4-tropic NL4.3 but not by CCR5-tropic p81.A (Figure 6 and Table S1).

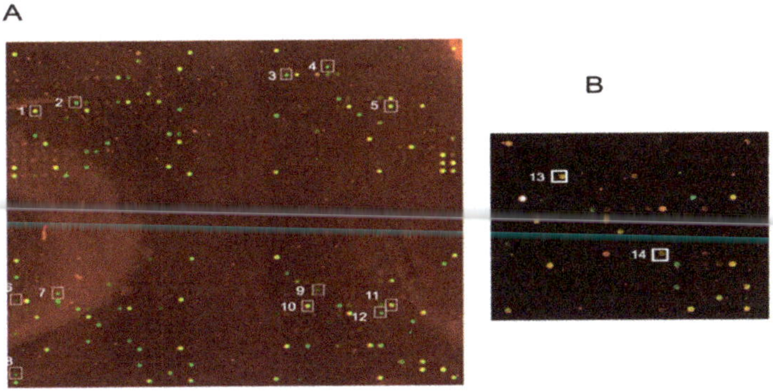

Figure 6. Photographs of arrays representing transcriptional changes in macrophages infected by 81A and NL4-3 strains. In array (**A**) the Cy3 spots indicated by numbered squares represent the apoptosis-related genes activated by NL4-3 whereas in subarray (**B**) the Cy5 spots indicated by numbered squares represent the survival-related genes activated by 81A. The square numbers relative to the genes are also indicated in Table S1.

4. Discussion

This study shows that CCR5-tropic and CXCR4-tropic strains exhibit different kinetics of replication in MDM and highlights the capability of CXCR4-tropic strains to promote the apoptosis of this important HIV-1 reservoir. HIV-1 reservoirs represent so far the major obstacle for achieving HIV cure.

Our findings are in line with a previous study showing that differences between CCR5-tropic strains and CXCR4 strains in productive infection of MDM occurred during the early stages of HIV-1 life cycle and in particles at levels of reverse transcription and nuclear translocation of viral genomes [32]. Though our study did not consider the phase22s of HIV life cycle, we investigated a relationship between different levels in viral production and MDM homeostasis according to co-receptor usage.

We evaluated different kinetics of replication in MDM of CXCR4-tropic and CCR5-tropic molecular clones, respectively, NL4-3 and 81A, differing only in env variable domains. After a starting boost, the replication of CXCR4-tropic clones in MDM subsequently diminished reaching a status of abortive infection, while the replication of CCR5-tropic clones tended to increase, reaching a plateau after 10 days of infection.

It is important to stress that NL4-3 did not affect HIV-1 productive infection up to the seventh day in MDM, suggesting that the clearance of the CXCR4 strain may not be due to a failure in the entry or in other preintegrational phases (Figure 1), but may be the result of the killing of the host cells during the onset of infection.

These results underline the tendency towards an in vitro disappearance of the most aggressive CXCR4- tropic virus in the course of the HIV-1 infection and the survival of CCR5- tropic strain infected MDM reservoirs as key determinant of HIV-1 persistence in this cellular reservoir.

This evidence provided us the clue to analyze how coreceptor usage may differently modulate MDM homeostasis and particularly apoptosis.

In particular, the MAPK p38 plays a pivotal role in the transmission of signals from cell surface receptors to the nucleus. It is activated by diverse extracellular stimuli that regulate important cellular processes including response to stress factors in many cell types [66]. Our results show a transient but marked induction of the phosphorylated form of the p38 MAPK at 30′ after exposure to CXCR4-tropic, but not CCR5-tropic HIV strains in MDM. The role of activation of MAPKs p38 in programmed death of MDM and T-cells due to CXCR4-tropic strain infection still remains controversial: whereas a role in HIV pathogenicity is already demonstrated [50,67], some studies report no association in Caspase-dependent apoptosis [68] moreover, the p38 activation pathway, in cell reservoirs such as MDM, was attributed to β chemokine secretion rather than apoptosis [49,69]. In this last case, this disagreement with our results in HIV mediated signalling may be attributed to a different experimental approach as we used the whole pure viruses and not the recombinant gp120 and did not consider any serum starvation for exposure of MDM to the different strains, in order to avoid them excessive stress and permit the primary cells to reproduce under more natural physiological conditions.

The role of p38 has been elucidated in the setting of infection of T cells by CXCR4-tropic strains [70,71]. In particular, the role of replication of HIV-1 in human T lymphocytes requires the activation of host cellular proteins [72]. Previous studies have identified p38 mitogen-activated protein kinase (MAPK) as a kinase necessary for HIV-1 replication in T cells [73–76]. Among them, Cohen et al. 1997 have shown that HIV-1 CXCR4 strain infection of both primary human T lymphocytes and T cell lines immediately stimulates the cellular p38 MAPK pathway, which remains activated throughout the experimental conditions. Inclusion of an antisense oligonucleotides to p38 MAPK expressly inhibited viral replication [70,77–79]. Blockade of p38 MAPK by addition of CNI-1493 also inhibited HIV-1 viral replication of primary T lymphocytes in a dose- and time-dependent manner. Stimulation of p38 MAPK activation did not occur with the addition of heat-inactivated virus, suggesting that viral internalization, and not just membrane binding, is necessary for p38 MAPK activation [80,81]. The results of this work show that activation of the p38 MAPK cascade is critical and essential for HIV-1 replication in T cells [81,82].

In consideration of key determinants of HIV persistence in MDM reservoirs, post translation changes of cell and nuclear targets is one of the upstream events due to viral exposure, culminating in absence of cytolitic effects. Macrophages provide an ideal environment for the formation of viral reservoirs since they live long and are widely distributed throughout the body [83].

As microarray analysis showed, 10 genes related to the apoptosis pathway were up-regulated in NL4-3 infected MDM compared to 81A infected ones and genes related to the apoptosis pathway, such as Defender against cell death 1(DAD-1) [84] and Cullin 2 (hCUL2), were up-regulated in 81A infected compared to NL4-3 infected MDM.

Our studies demonstrate the up-regulation of genes included the polypeptide chain-releasing factor GSPT1/eRF3 protein, which in the processed form has been shown to promote caspase activation, IAP (inhibitors of apoptosis) ubiquitination and apoptosis [53], Caspase 7 (CASP 7), an apoptosis-related [69] and Cytochrome C whose release has been shown in HIV dependent apoptosis [50]. The activation of such genes related to apoptosis in NL4-3 infected MDM can then have downstream effects being responsible for the progressive decrease of p24 production of the CXCR4-using NL4.3.

Our results would not seem in line with in vivo evidence of the emergence of the more aggressive sincytium-inducing (SI) CXCR4- tropic strains in the terminal phases of HIV-1 disease associated with rapid decline of CD4+ and CD8+ T cells [28,85] but this phenomenon almost represents an effect of the breakdown of the immune system and the onset of AIDS [86]. We speculate that CXCR4- tropic strains play a minor role in disease progression because dying CXCR4 virus infected reservoirs, cannot provide virus nor continue to directly contribute to the depletion of immune cell system. Indeed, CCR5-using strains are associated with a lower percentage of cell death, suggesting the capability of these strains to promote cell survival as supported also by transcriptome analysis.

On the other hand, there are many reasons to consider a role of CCR5 viruses and their host cells as target for therapeutic strategies: (i) the protective role of the 32-nucleotides (Δ32) deletion in CCR5 gene in homozygous condition against HIV-1 infection and the more benign pattern of disease progression associated with the deletion in one of the two alleles [87,88] (ii) a logarithmic correlation between CCR5 expression and viremia in patients with disease progression [89–91] (iii) the importance of CCR5-tropic isolates for dissemination outside peripheral blood in compartments considered as "sanctuaries" like the Central Nervous System where macrophages represent more than 90% of the

HIV-1 infected cells [92–95] the capacity of R5 isolates harbored in macrophagic reservoirs to provoke the immune anergy through host-related factors (bystander effect) and the emergence of more virulent SI variants and the subsequent AIDS progression (iv) increase of viremia in later stages of HIV disease caused by macrophages during opportunistic infections [96,97] (v) increase of both CCR5 expression on CD4+ T cells and the frequency of memory CD4 T-cells (the target cells of CCR5 virus variants) over the course of infection [97,98].

5. Conclusions

To summarize, CCR5 strains induce chronic and productive infection in MDM whereas CXCR4-tropic strains induce abortive infection. Moreover, the abrogation of HIV-1-dependent killing due to the specific CXCR4 inhibitor AMD3100 indicates the obligatory role of CXCR4. Phosphorylation of p38 (MAP Kinase family), reported to be activated after exposure to many forms of cellular stress, is enhanced by the CXCR4-tropic strain NL4-3 and IIIB and not by CCR5-tropic strain 81A and BaL; also, this induction is modulated by CXCR4. CXCR4-tropic strains activate inflammatory genes in MDM whereas CCR5-tropic HIV-1 strains do not induce a death program in MDM.

Taken together, our results correlate with in vitro and in vivo evidence about an uncoupling between viral replication and cytopathocity [88] and confirm what we observed previously [9,99] in later phases of infection: MDM homeostasis is up-regulated where infection is sustained by CCR5-tropic strains. All the CXCR4-tropic strains we used, in contrast, induce MDM apoptosis and lead to consequent clearance of HIV replication. Further studies are necessary to investigate if gp120 interaction with CXCR4 in MDM can also induce the activation of pro-inflammatory pathways.

Our findings provide important implications for HIV-1 pathogenesis and design of pharmacological targets aimed at achieving HIV-1 cure.

Supplementary Materials: The following are available online at http://www.mdpi.com/1010-660X/55/6/297/s1, Table S1: Different changes in genes in R5 virus versus X4 virus-infected incubated MDM.

Author Contributions: S.A. and C.F.P. conceived of and designed the experiments. A.R., M.P., M.C.B. and R.S. performed the experiments. A.B., A.R., V.S. and S.A. analyzed the data. M.C.B., M.V.M. and F.C.-S. contributed reagents, materials, and analysis tools. A.B., A.R., V.S. and S.A. wrote the paper.

Acknowledgments: Authors would like to thank D. Schols for providing both antiviral compounds and clinical isolates. This work was supported by PRIN (Progetti di Rilevante Interesse Nazionale) Grant 2015W729WH_007 and 2017M8R7N9_004 from the MIUR, Italy and by GAIN (Agencia Gallega de Innovación) Grant IN606B-2016/012 from the Consellería de Cultura, Educación e Ordenación Universitaria e a Consellería de Economía, Emprego e Industria (Xunta de Galicia), Spain.

Conflicts of Interest: The authors declare no conflict of interest.

References

1. Richman, D.D.; Margolis, D.M.; Delaney, M.; Greene, W.C.; Hazuda, D.; Pomerantz, R.J. The challenge of finding a cure for HIV infection. *Science* **2009**, *323*, 1304–1307. [CrossRef] [PubMed]
2. International AIDS Society Scientific Working Group on HIV Cure; Deeks, S.G.; Autran, B.; Berkhout, B.; Benkirane, M.; Cairns, S.; Chomont, N.; Chun, T.W.; Churchill, M.; Di Mascio, M.; et al. Towards an HIV cure: A global scientific strategy. *Nat. Rev. Immunol.* **2012**, *12*, 607–614. [PubMed]
3. Ramratnam, B.; Mittler, J.E.; Zhang, L.; Boden, D.; Hurley, A.; Fang, F.; Macken, C.A.; Perelson, A.S.; Markowitz, M.; Ho, D.D. The decay of the latent reservoir of replication-competent HIV-1 is inversely correlated with the extent of residual viral replication during prolonged anti-retroviral therapy. *Nat. Med.* **2000**, *6*, 82–85. [CrossRef] [PubMed]
4. Borrajo, A.; Ranazzi, A.; Pollicita, M.; Bruno, R.; Modesti, A.; Alteri, C.; Perno, C.F.; Svicher, V.; Aquaro, S. Effects of Amprenavir on HIV-1 Maturation, Production and Infectivity Following Drug Withdrawal in Chronically-Infected Monocytes/Macrophages. *Viruses* **2017**, *9*, 277. [CrossRef] [PubMed]
5. Crowe, S.M.; Sonza, S. HIV-1 can be recovered from a variety of cells including peripheral blood monocytes of patients receiving highly active antiretroviral therapy: A further obstacle to eradication. *J. Leukoc. Biol.* **2000**, *68*, 345–350. [PubMed]

6. Kulpa, D.A.; Chomont, N. HIV persistence in the setting of antiretroviral therapy: When, where and how does HIV hide? *J. Virus Erad.* **2015**, *1*, 59–66. [PubMed]
7. Perno, C.F.; Yarchoan, R.; Cooney, D.A.; Hartman, N.R.; Webb, D.S.; Hao, Z.; Mitsuya, H.; Johns, D.G.; Broder, S. Replication of human immunodeficiency virus in monocytes. Granulocyte/macrophage colony-stimulating factor (GM-CSF) potentiates viral production yet enhances the antiviral effect mediated by 3′-azido-2′3′-dideoxythymidine (AZT) and other dideoxynucleoside congeners of thymidine. *J. Exp. Med.* **1989**, *169*, 933–951. [PubMed]
8. Whal, S.M.; Greenwell-Wild, T.; Peng, G.; Ma, G.; Orenstein, J.M.; Vasquez, N. Viral and host cofactors facilitate HIV-1 replication in macrophages. *J. Leukoc.* **2003**, *74*, 726–735. [CrossRef] [PubMed]
9. Aquaro, S.; Bagnarelli, P.; Guenci, T.; De Luca, A.; Clementi, M.; Balestra, E.; Caliò, R.; Perno, C.F. Long-term survival and virus production in Human Primary Macrophages infected by Human Immunodeficiency Virus. *J. Med. Virol.* **2002**, *68*, 479–488. [CrossRef] [PubMed]
10. Collman, R.G.; Perno, C.F.; Crowe, S.M.; Stevenson, M.; Montaner, L.J. HIV and cells of macrophage/dendritic lineage and other non-T cell reservoirs: New answers yield new questions. *J. Leukoc. Biol.* **2003**, *74*, 631–634. [CrossRef]
11. Deng, K.; Siliciano, R.F. HIV: Early treatment may not be early enough. *Nature* **2014**, *512*, 35–36. [CrossRef] [PubMed]
12. Van Lint, C.; Bouchat, S.; Marcello, A. HIV-1 transcription and latency: An update. *Retrovirology* **2013**, *10*, 67. [CrossRef] [PubMed]
13. Hong, F.F.; Mellors, J.W. Changes in HIV reservoirs during long-term antiretroviral therapy. *Curr. Opin. HIV AIDS* **2015**, *10*, 43–48. [CrossRef] [PubMed]
14. Siliciano, R.F. Opening Fronts in HIV Vaccine Development: Targeting reservoirs to clear and cure. *Nat. Med.* **2014**, *20*, 480–481. [CrossRef] [PubMed]
15. Abbas, W.; Tariq, M.; Iqbal, M.; Kumar, A.; Herbein, G. Eradication of HIV-1 from the Macrophage Reservoir: An Uncertain Goal. *Viruses* **2015**, *7*, 1578–1598. [CrossRef] [PubMed]
16. Lv, Z.; Chu, Y.; Wang, Y. HIV protease inhibitors: A review of molecular selectivity and toxicity. *HIV AIDS* **2015**, *7*, 95–104.
17. Merino, K.M.; Allers, C.; Didier, E.S.; Kuroda, M.J. Role of Monocyte/Macrophages during HIV/SIV Infection in Adult and Pediatric Acquired Immune Deficiency Syndrome. *Front. Immunol.* **2017**, *8*, 1693. [CrossRef]
18. Vanham, G.; Penne, L.; Allemeersch, H.; Kestens, L.; Willems, B.; van der Groen, G.; Jeang, K.T.; Toossi, Z.; Rich, E. Modeling HIV transfer between dendritic cells and T cells: Importance of HIV phenotype, dendritic cell-T cell contact and T-cell activation. *AIDS* **2000**, *14*, 2299–2311. [CrossRef]
19. Klatzmann, D.; Champagne, E.; Chamaret, S.; Gruest, J.; Guetard, D.; Hercend, T.; Gluckman, J.C.; Montagnier, L. T-Lymphocyte T4 molecule behaves as receptor for human retrovirus LA.V. *Nature* **1984**, *312*, 767–768. [CrossRef]
20. Durham, N.D.; Chen, B.K. Measuring T Cell-to-T Cell HIV-1 Transfer, Viral Fusion, and Infection Using Flow Cytometry. *Methods Mol. Biol.* **2016**, *1354*, 21–38.
21. Quitadamo, B.; Peters, P.J.; Repik, A.; O'Connell, O.; Mou, Z.; Koch, M.; Somasundaran, M.; Brody, R.; Luzuriaga, K.; Wallace, A.; et al. HIV-1 R5 Macrophage-Tropic Envelope Glycoprotein Trimers Bind CD4 with High Affinity, while the CD4 Binding Site on Non-macrophage-tropic, T-Tropic R5 Envelopes Is Occluded. *J. Virol.* **2018**, *92*, e00841-17. [CrossRef] [PubMed]
22. Petrov, V.; Funderburg, N.; Weinberg, A.; Sieg, S. Human β defensin-3 induces chemokines from monocytes and macrophages: Diminished activity in cells from HIV-infected persons. *Immunology* **2013**, *140*, 413–420. [CrossRef] [PubMed]
23. Wang, H.W.; Zhu, B.; Hou, L.J.; Lu, G.J.; Jiao, L.Y.; Shen, B.S. An infectious molecular clone in early infection with HIV-1 subtype CRF01_AE strains: Construction and biological properties. *Mol. Biol. Rep.* **2015**, *42*, 329–336. [CrossRef] [PubMed]
24. Bolduc, J.F.; Ouellet, M.; Hany, L.; Tremblay, M.J. Toll-Like Receptor 2 Ligation Enhances HIV-1 Replication in Activated CCR6+ CD4+ T Cells by Increasing Virus Entry and Establishing a More Permissive Environment to Infection. *J. Virol.* **2017**, *91*, e01402-16. [CrossRef] [PubMed]
25. Willey, S.; Peters, P.J.; Sullivan, W.M.; Dorr, P.; Perros, M.; Clapham, P.R. Inhibition of CCR5-mediated infection by diverse R5 and R5X4 HIV and SIV isolates using novel small molecule inhibitors of CCR5: Effects of viral diversity, target cell and receptor density. *Antivir. Res.* **2005**, *68*, 96–108. [CrossRef] [PubMed]

26. Nixon, D.F. R5 human immunodeficiency virus type 1 (HIV-1) replicates more efficiently in primary CD4+ T-cell cultures than X4 HIV-1. *J. Virol.* **2004**, *78*, 9164–9173.
27. Feng, Y.; Broder, C.C.; Kennedy, P.E.; Berger, E.A. Pillars article: HIV-1 entry cofactor: Functional cDNA cloning of a seven-transmembrane, G protein-coupled receptor. *J. Immunol.* **2011**, *186*, 6076–6081. [PubMed]
28. Kwa, D.; Vingerhoed, J.; Boeser-Nunnink, B.; Broersen, S.; Schuitemaker, H. Cytopathic Effects of Non-Syncytium-Inducing and Syncytium-Inducing Human Immunodeficiency Virus Type 1 Variants on Different CD4+-T-Cell Subsets Are Determined Only by Coreceptor Expression. *J. Virol.* **2001**, *75*, 10455–10459. [CrossRef] [PubMed]
29. Upadhyay, C.; Feyznezhad, R.; Yang, W.; Zhang, H.; Zolla-Pazner, S.; Hioe, C.E. Alterations of HIV-1 envelope phenotype and antibody-mediated neutralization by signal peptide mutations. *PLoS Pathog.* **2018**, *14*, e1006812. [CrossRef]
30. Yi, Y.; Singh, A.; Isaacs, S.N.; Collman, R.G. A CCR5/CXCR4-independent coreceptor pathway on human macrophages supports efficient SIV env-mediated fusion but not infection: Implications for alternative pathways of viral entry. *Virology* **2001**, *284*, 142–151. [CrossRef]
31. Gorry, P.R.; Ancuta, P. Coreceptors and HIV-1 pathogenesis. *Curr. HIV AIDS Rep.* **2011**, *8*, 45–53. [CrossRef] [PubMed]
32. Gorry, P.R.; Bristol, G.; Zack, J.A.; Ritola, K.; Swanstrom, R.; Birch, C.J.; Bell, J.E.; Bannert, N.; Crawford, K.; Wang, H.; et al. Macrophage tropism of human immunodeficiency virus type 1 isolates from brain and lymphoid tissues predicts neurotropism independent of coreceptor specificity. *J. Virol.* **2001**, *75*, 10073–10089. [CrossRef] [PubMed]
33. Gray, L.; Sterjovski, J.; Churchill, M.; Ellery, P.; Nasr, N.; Lewin, S.R.; Crowe, S.M.; Wesselingh, S.L.; Cunningham, A.L.; Gorry, P.R. Uncoupling coreceptor usage of human immunodeficiency virus type 1 (HIV-1) from macrophage tropism reveals biological properties of CCR5-restricted HIV-1 isolates from patients with acquired immunodeficiency syndrome. *Virology* **2005**, *337*, 384–398. [CrossRef] [PubMed]
34. Isaacman-Beck, J.; Hermann, E.A.; Yi, Y.; Ratcliffe, S.J.; Mulenga, J.; Allen, S.; Hunter, E.; Derdeyn, C.A.; Collman, R.G. Heterosexual transmission of human immunodeficiency virus type 1 subtype C: Macrophage tropism, alternative coreceptor use, and the molecular anatomy of CCR5 utilization. *J. Virol.* **2009**, *83*, 8208–8220. [CrossRef] [PubMed]
35. Peters, P.J.; Bhattacharya, J.; Hibbitts, S.; Dittmar, M.T.; Simmons, G.; Bell, J.; Simmonds, P.; Clapham, P.R. Biological analysis of human immunodeficiency virus type 1 R5 envelopes amplified from brain and lymph node tissues of AIDS patients with neuropathology reveals two distinct tropism phenotypes and identifies envelopes in the brain that confer an enhanced tropism and fusigenicity for macrophages. *J. Virol.* **2004**, *78*, 6915–6926. [PubMed]
36. Peters, P.J.; Duenas-Decamp, M.J.; Sullivan, W.M.; Brown, R.; Ankghuambom, C.; Luzuriaga, K.; Robinson, J.; Burton, D.R.; Bell, J.; Simmonds, P.; et al. Variation in HIV-1 R5 macrophage-tropism correlates with sensitivity to reagents that block envelope: CD4 interactions but not with sensitivity to other entry inhibitors. *Retrovirology* **2008**, *5*, 5. [CrossRef]
37. Peters, P.J.; Sullivan, W.M.; Duenas-Decamp, M.J.; Bhattacharya, J.; Ankghuambom, C.; Brown, R.; Luzuriaga, K.; Bell, J.; Simmonds, P.; Ball, J.; et al. Non-macrophage-tropic human immunodeficiency virus type 1 R5 envelopes predominate in blood, lymph nodes, and semen: Implications for transmission and pathogenesis. *J. Virol.* **2006**, *80*, 6324–6332. [CrossRef]
38. Cashin, K.; Roche, M.; Sterjovski, J.; Ellett, A.; Gray, L.R.; Cunningham, A.L.; Ramsland, P.A.; Churchill, M.J.; Gorry, P.R. Alternative Coreceptor Requirements for Efficient CCR5- and CXCR4-Mediated HIV-1 Entry into Macrophages. *J. Virol.* **2011**, *85*, 10699–10709. [CrossRef]
39. Kumar, A.; Herbein, G. The macrophage: A therapeutic target in HIV-1 infection. *Mol. Cell. Ther.* **2014**, *2*, 10. [CrossRef]
40. Berro, R.; de la Fuente, C.; Klase, Z.; Kehn, K.; Parvin, L.; Pumfery, A.; Agbottah, E.; Vertes, A.; Nekhai, S.; Kashanchi, F. Identifying the membrane proteome of HIV-1 latently infected cells. *J. Biol. Chem.* **2007**, *282*, 8207–8218. [CrossRef]
41. Tan, J.; Wang, X.; Devadas, K.; Zhao, J.; Zhang, P.; Hewlett, I. Some mechanisms of FLIP expression in inhibition of HIV-1 replication in Jurkat cells, CD4+T cells and PBMCs. *J. Cell. Physiol.* **2013**, *228*, 2305–2313. [CrossRef] [PubMed]

42. Timilsina, U.; Gaur, R. Modulation of apoptosis and viral latency—An axis to be well understood for successful cure of human immunodeficiency virus. *J. Gen. Virol.* **2016**, *97*, 813–824. [CrossRef] [PubMed]
43. Badley, A.D.; Sainski, A.; Wightman, F.; Lewin, S.R. Altering cell death pathways as an approach to cure HIV infection. *Cell Death Dis.* **2013**, *4*, e718. [CrossRef] [PubMed]
44. Wang, X.; Ragupathy, V.; Zhao, J.; Hewlett, I. Molecules from apoptotic pathways modulate HIV-1 replication in Jurkat cells. *Biochem. Biophys. Res. Commun.* **2011**, *414*, 20–24. [CrossRef] [PubMed]
45. Jones, A.T.; Chamcha, V.; Kesavardhana, S.; Shen, X.; Beaumont, D.; Das, R.; Wyatt, L.S.; LaBranche, C.C.; Stanfield-Oakley, S.; Ferrari, G.; et al. A trimeric HIV-1 envelope gp120 immunogen induces potent and broad anti-V1V2 loop antibodies against HIV-1 in rabbits and rhesus macaques. *J. Virol.* **2017**, *92*, e01796-17. [CrossRef] [PubMed]
46. Gartner, S.; Markovits, P.; Markovitz, D.M.; Kaplan, M.H.; Gallo, R.C.; Popovic, M. The role of Mononuclear phagocytes in HTLV-III/LAV infection. *Science* **1986**, *233*, 215–219. [CrossRef] [PubMed]
47. Cenci, A.; Perno, C.F.; Menzo, S.; Clementi, M.; Erba, F.; Tavazzi, B.; Di Pierro, D.; Aquaro, S.; Calio, R. Selected nucleotide sequence of the pol gene of the monocytotropic strain HIV type 1 BaL. *AIDS Res. Hum. Retrovir.* **1997**, *13*, 629–632. [CrossRef] [PubMed]
48. Knight, J.C.; Hallett, A.J.; Brancale, A.; Paisey, S.J.; Clarkson, R.W.; Edwards, P.G. Evaluation of a fluorescent derivative of AMD3100 and its interaction with the CXCR4 chemokine receptor. *ChemBioChem* **2011**, *12*, 2692–2698. [CrossRef] [PubMed]
49. Foster, T.L.; Pickering, S.; Neil, S.J.D. Inhibiting the Ins and Outs of HIV Replication: Cell-Intrinsic Antiretroviral Restrictions at the Plasma Membrane. *Front. Immunol.* **2018**, *8*, 1853. [CrossRef]
50. Saiman, Y.; Jiao, J.; Fiel, M.I.; Friedman, S.L.; Aloman, C.; Bansal, M.B. Inhibition of the CXCL12/CXCR4 chemokine axis with AMD3100, a CXCR4 small molecule inhibitor, worsens murine hepatic injury. *Hepatol. Res.* **2015**, *45*, 794–803. [CrossRef]
51. Shiraishi, M.; Aramaki, Y.; Seto, M.; Imoto, H.; Nishikawa, Y.; Kanzaki, N.; Okamoto, M.; Sawada, H.; Nishimura, O.; Baba, M.; et al. Discovery of novel, potent, and selective small-molecule CCR5 antagonists as anti-HIV-1 agents: Synthesis and biological evaluation of anilide derivatives with a quaternary ammonium moiety. *J. Med. Chem.* **2000**, *43*, 2049–2063. [CrossRef] [PubMed]
52. Paterlini, M.G. Structure modeling of the chemokine receptor CCR5: Implications for ligand binding and selectivity. *Biophys. J.* **2002**, *83*, 3012–3031. [CrossRef]
53. Regoes, R.R.; Bonhoeffer, S. The HIV coreceptor switch: A population dynamical perspective. *Trends Microbiol.* **2005**, *13*, 269–277. [CrossRef] [PubMed]
54. Bakri, Y.; Mannioui, A.; Ylisastigui, L.; Sanchez, F.; Gluckman, J.C.; Benjouad, A. CD40-activated macrophages become highly susceptible to X4 strains of human immunodeficiency virus type 1. *AIDS Res. Hum. Retrovir.* **2002**, *18*, 103–113. [CrossRef] [PubMed]
55. Nagata, S.; Imai, J.; Makino, G.; Tomita, M.; Kanai, A. Evolutionary Analysis of HIV-1 Pol Proteins Reveals Representative Residues for Viral Subtype Differentiation. *Front. Microbiol.* **2017**, *8*, 2151. [CrossRef] [PubMed]
56. Council, O.D.; Joseph, S.B. Evolution of Host Target Cell Specificity During HIV-1 Infection. *Curr. HIV Res.* **2017**, *16*, 13–20. [CrossRef] [PubMed]
57. Naif, H.M. Pathogenesis of HIV Infection. *Infect. Dis. Rep.* **2013**, *5* (Suppl. 1), e6. [CrossRef] [PubMed]
58. Naif, H.M.; Cunningham, A.L.; Alali, M.; Li, S.; Nasr, N.; Buhler, M.M.; Schols, D.; de Clercq, E.; Stewart, G. A human immunodeficiency virus type 1 isolate from an infected person homozygous for CCR5Delta32 exhibits dual tropism by infecting macrophages and MT2 cells via CXCR4. *J. Virol.* **2002**, *76*, 3114–3124. [CrossRef] [PubMed]
59. Princen, K.; Hatse, S.; Vermeire, K.; Aquaro, S.; De Clercq, E.; Gerlach, L.O.; Rosenkilde, M.; Schwartz, T.W.; Skerlj, R.; Bridger, G.; et al. Inhibition of human immunodeficiency virus replication by a dual CCR5/CXCR4 antagonist. *J. Virol.* **2004**, *78*, 12996–13006. [CrossRef]
60. Bagnarelli, P.; Valenza, A.; Menzo, S.; Sampaollesi, R.; Varaldo, P.E.; Butini, L.; Montoni, M.; Perno, C.F.; Aquaro, S.; Mathez, D.; et al. Dynamics and modulation of Human Immunodeficency virus type I transcripts in vitro and in vivo. *J. Virol.* **1996**, *70*, 7603–7613.
61. Baxter, A.E.; Niessl, J.; Morou, A.; Kaufmann, D.E. RNA flow cytometric FISH for investigations into HIV immunology, vaccination and cure strategies. *AIDS Res. Ther.* **2017**, *14*, 40. [CrossRef] [PubMed]

62. Perfettini, J.L.; Castedo, M.; Nardacci, R.; Ciccosanti, F.; Boya, P.; Roumier, T.; Larochette, N.; Piacentini, M.; Kroemer, G. Essential role of p53 phosphorylation by p38 MAPK in apoptosis induction by the HIV-1 envelope. *J. Exp. Med.* **2005**, *201*, 279–289. [CrossRef] [PubMed]
63. Trinklein, N.D.; Chen, W.C.; Kingston, R.E.; Myers, R.M. Transcriptional regulation and binding of heat shock factor 1 and heat shock factor 2 to 32 human heat shock genes during thermal stress and differentiation. *Cell Stress Chaperones* **2004**, *9*, 21–28. [CrossRef]
64. Fehrenbach, H.; Kasper, M.; Koslowski, R.; Pan, T.; Schuh, D.; Muller, M.; Mason, R.J. Alveolar epithelial type II cell apoptosis in vivo during resolution of keratinocyte growth factor-induced hyperplasia in the rat. *Histochem. Cell Biol.* **2000**, *114*, 49–61. [PubMed]
65. Hegde, R.; Srinivasula, S.M.; Datta, P.; Madesh, M.; Wassell, R.; Zhang, Z.; Cheong, N.; Nejmeh, J.; Fernandes-Alnemri, T.; Hoshino, S.; et al. The polypeptide chain-releasing factor GSPT1/eRF3 is proteolytically processed into an IAP-binding protein. *J. Biol. Chem.* **2003**, *278*, 38699–38706. [CrossRef] [PubMed]
66. Herbein, G.; Gras, G.; Khan, K.A.; Abbas, W. Macrophage signaling in HIV-1 infection. *Retrovirology* **2010**, *7*, 34. [CrossRef]
67. Kumar, A.; Abbas, W.; Herbein, G. TNF and TNF receptor superfamily members in HIV infection: New cellular targets for therapy? *Mediat. Inflamm.* **2013**, *2013*, 484378. [CrossRef]
68. Ahr, B.; Robert-Hebmann, V.; Devaux, C.; Biard-Piechaczyk, M. Apoptosis of uninfected cells induced by HIV envelope glycoproteins. *Retrovirology* **2004**, *1*, 12. [CrossRef]
69. Espert, L.; Denizot, M.; Grimaldi, M.; Robert-Hebmann, V.; Gay, B.; Varbanov, M.; Codogno, P.; Biard-Piechaczyk, M. Autophagy is involved in T cell death after binding of HIV-1 envelope proteins to CXCR4. *J. Clin. Investig.* **2006**, *116*, 2161–2172. [CrossRef]
70. Cohen, P.S.; Schmidtmayerova, H.; Dennis, J.; Dubrovsky, L.; Sherry, B.; Wang, H.; Bukrinsky, M.; Tracey, K.J. The critical role of p38 MAP kinase in T cell HIV-1 replication. *Mol. Med.* **1997**, *3*, 339–346. [CrossRef]
71. Kralova, J.; Dvorak, M.; Koc, M.; Kral, V. p38 MAPK plays an essential role in apoptosis induced by photoactivation of a novel ethylene glycol porphyrin derivative. *Oncogene* **2008**, *27*, 3010–3020. [CrossRef] [PubMed]
72. Bai, L.; Zhu, X.; Ma, T.; Wang, J.; Wang, F.; Zhang, S. The p38 MAPK NF-κB pathway, not the ERK pathway, is involved in exogenous HIV-1 Tat-induced apoptotic cell death in retinal pigment epithelial cells. *Int. J. Biochem. Cell Biol.* **2013**, *45*, 1794–1801. [CrossRef] [PubMed]
73. Petrovas, C.; Mueller, Y.M.; Katsikis, P.D. Apoptosis of HIV-specific CD8+ T cells:an HIV evasion strategy. *Cell Death Differ.* **2005**, *12* (Suppl. 1), 859–870. [CrossRef] [PubMed]
74. Blanco, J.; Barretina, J.; Henson, G.; Bridger, G.; De Clercq, E.; Clotet, B.; Este, J.A. The CXCR4 antagonist AMD3100 efficiently inhibits cell-surface-expressed human immunodeficiency virus type 1 envelope-induced apoptosis. *Antimicrob. Agents Chemother.* **2000**, *44*, 51–56. [CrossRef] [PubMed]
75. Checkley, M.A.; Luttge, B.G.; Freed, E.O. HIV-1 envelope glycoprotein biosynthesis, trafficking, and incorporation. *J. Mol. Biol.* **2011**, *410*, 582–608. [CrossRef] [PubMed]
76. Gougeon, M.L.; Chiodi, F. Impact of gamma-chain cytokines on T cell homeostasis in HIV-1 infection: Therapeutic implications. *J. Intern. Med.* **2010**, *267*, 502–514. [CrossRef] [PubMed]
77. Wang, J.; Crawford, K.; Yuan, M.; Wang, H.; Gorry, P.R.; Gabuzda, D. Regulation of CC chemokine receptor 5 and CD4 expression and human immunodeficiency virus type 1 replication in human macrophages and microglia by T helper type 2 cytokines. *J. Infect. Dis.* **2002**, *185*, 885–897. [CrossRef] [PubMed]
78. Kim, H.Y.; Hwang, J.Y.; Oh, Y.S.; Kim, S.W.; Lee, H.J.; Yun, H.J.; Kim, S.; Yang, Y.J.; Jo, D.Y. Differential effects of CXCR4 antagonists on the survival and proliferation of myeloid leukemia cells in vitro. *Korean J. Hematol.* **2011**, *46*, 244–252. [CrossRef] [PubMed]
79. Singhal, P.C.; Bhaskaran, M.; Patel, J.; Patel, K.; Kasinath, B.S.; Duraisamy, S.; Franki, N.; Reddy, K.; Kapasi, A.A. Role of p38 mitogen-activated protein kinase phosphorylation and Fas-Fas ligand interaction in morphine-induced macrophage apoptosis. *J. Immunol.* **2002**, *168*, 4025–4033. [CrossRef]
80. Muthumani, K.; Wadsworth, S.A.; Dayes, N.S.; Hwang, D.S.; Choo, A.Y.; Abeysinghe, H.R.; Siekierka, J.J.; Weiner, D.B. Suppression of HIV-1 viral replication and cellular pathogenesis by a novel p38/JNK kinase inhibitor. *AIDS* **2004**, *18*, 739–748. [CrossRef]

81. Biard-Piechaczyk, M.; Robert-Hebmann, V.; Richard, V.; Roland, J.; Hipskind, R.A.; Devaux, C. Caspase-dependent apoptosis of cells expressing the chemokine receptor CXCR4 is induced by cell membrane-associated human immunodeficiency virus type 1 envelope glycoprotein (gp120). *Virology* **2000**, *268*, 329–344. [CrossRef] [PubMed]
82. Hong, N.A.; Flannery, M.; Hsieh, S.N.; Cado, D.; Pedersen, R.; Winoto, A. Mice lacking Dad1, the defender against apoptotic death-1, express abnormal N-linked glycoproteins and undergo increased embryonic apoptosis. *Dev. Biol.* **2000**, *220*, 76–84. [CrossRef] [PubMed]
83. Kariya, R.; Taura, M.; Suzu, S.; Kai, H.; Katano, H.; Okada, S. HIV protease inhibitor Lopinavir induces apoptosis of primary effusion lymphoma cells via suppression of NF-κB pathway. *Cancer Lett.* **2014**, *342*, 52–59. [CrossRef] [PubMed]
84. Garrido, C.; Kroemer, G. Life's smile, death's grin: Vital functions of apoptosis-executing proteins. *Curr. Opin. Cell Biol.* **2004**, *16*, 639–646. [CrossRef] [PubMed]
85. Lin, N.; Gonzalez, O.A.; Registre, L.; Becerril, C.; Etemad, B.; Lu, H.; Wu, X.; Lockman, S.; Essex, M.; Moyo, S.; et al. Humoral Immune Pressure Selects for HIV-1 CXC-chemokine Receptor 4-using Variants. *EBioMedicine* **2016**, *8*, 237–247. [CrossRef] [PubMed]
86. Svicher, V.; Marchetti, G.; Ammassari, A.; Ceccherini-Silberstein, F.; Sarmati, L. Impact Study Group. Novelties in Evaluation and Monitoring of Human Immunodeficiency Virus-1 Infection: Is Standard Virological Suppression Enoughfor Measuring Antiretroviral Treatment Success? *AIDS Rev.* **2017**, *19*, 119–133. [CrossRef] [PubMed]
87. Singh, H.; Samani, D.; Ghate, M.V.; Gangakhedkar, R.R. Impact of cellular restriction gene (TRIM5α, BST-2) polymorphisms on the acquisition of HIV-1 and disease progression. *J. Gene Med.* **2018**, *20*, e3004. [CrossRef]
88. Poropatich, K.; Sullivan, D.J., Jr. Human immunodeficiency virus type 1 long-term non-progressors: The viral, genetic and immunological basis for disease non-progression. *J. Gen. Virol.* **2011**, *92 Pt 2*, 247–268. [CrossRef]
89. Reynes, J.; Portales, P.; Segondy, M.; Baillat, V.; Andre, P.; Avinens, O.; Picot, M.C.; Clot, J.; Eliaou, J.F.; Corbeau, P. CD4 T cell surface CCR5 density as a host factor in HIV-1 disease progression. *AIDS* **2001**, *15*, 1627–1634. [CrossRef]
90. Reynes, J.; Portales, P.; Segondy, M.; Baillat, V.; Andre, P.; Reant, B.; Avinens, O.; Couderc, G.; Benkirane, M.; Clot, J.; et al. CD4+ T cell surface CCR5 density as a determining factor of virus load in persons infected with human immunodeficiency virus type 1. *J. Infect. Dis.* **2000**, *181*, 927–932. [CrossRef]
91. Kaul, M.; Garden, G.A.; Lipton, S.A. Pathways to neuronal injury and apoptosis in HIV-associated dementia. *Nature* **2001**, *410*, 988–994. [CrossRef] [PubMed]
92. Gonzalez-Perez, M.P.; Peters, P.J.; O'Connell, O.; Silva, N.; Harbison, C.; Cummings-Macri, S.; Kaliyaperumal, S.; Luzuriaga, K.; Clapham, P.R. Identification of Emerging Macrophage-Tropic HIV-1 R5 Variants in Brain Tissue of AIDS Patients without Severe Neurological Complications. *J. Virol.* **2017**, *91*, e00755-17. [CrossRef] [PubMed]
93. Lee, C.; Liu, Q.H.; Tomkowicz, B.; Yi, Y.; Freedman, B.D.; Collman, R.G. Macrophage activation through CCR5- and CXCR4-mediated gp120-elicited signaling pathways. *J. Leukoc. Biol.* **2003**, *74*, 676–682. [CrossRef] [PubMed]
94. Ashokkumar, M.; Nesakumar, M.; Cheedarla, N.; Vidyavijayan, K.K.; Babu, H.; Tripathy, S.P.; Hanna, L.E. Molecular Characteristics of the Envelope of Vertically Transmitted HIV-1 Strains from Infants with HIV Infection. *AIDS Res. Hum. Retrovir.* **2017**, *33*, 796–806. [CrossRef] [PubMed]
95. Avalos, C.R.; Abreu, C.M.; Queen, S.E.; Li, M.; Price, S.; Shirk, E.N.; Engle, E.L.; Forsyth, E.; Bullock, B.T.; Mac Gabhann, F.; et al. Brain Macrophages in Simian Immunodeficiency Virus-Infected, Antiretroviral-Suppressed Macaques: A Functional Latent Reservoir. *MBio* **2017**, *8*, e01186-17. [CrossRef] [PubMed]
96. Sebastian, N.T.; Zaikos, T.D.; Terry, V.; Taschuk, F.; McNamara, L.A.; Onafuwa-Nuga, A.; Yucha, R.; Signer, R.A.J.; Riddell, J., IV; Bixby, D.; et al. CD4 is expressed on a heterogeneous subset of hematopoietic progenitors, which persistently harbor CXCR4 and CCR5-tropic HIV proviral genomes in vivo. *PLoS Pathog.* **2017**, *13*, e1006509. [CrossRef]
97. Sandhu, A.; Ahmad, S.; Kaur, P.; Bhatnagar, A.; Dhawan, V.; Dhir, V. Methotrexate preferentially affects Tc1 and Tc17 subset of CD8 T lymphocytes. *Clin. Rheumatol.* **2019**, *38*, 37–44. [CrossRef] [PubMed]

98. Keppler, O.T.; Welte, F.J.; Ngo, T.A.; Chin, P.S.; Patton, K.S.; Tsou, C.L.; Abbey, N.W.; Sharkey, M.E.; Grant, R.M.; You, Y.; et al. Progress toward a human CD4/CCR5 transgenic rat model for de novo infection by human immunodeficiency virus type 1. *J. Exp. Med.* **2002**, *195*, 719–736. [CrossRef]
99. Garaci, E.; Caroleo, M.C.; Aloe, L.; Aquaro, S.; Piacentini, M.; Costa, N.; Amendola, A.; Micera, A.; Calio, R.; Perno, C.F.; et al. Nerve growth factor is an autocrine factor essential for the survival of macrophages infected with HIV. *Proc. Natl. Acad. Sci. USA* **1999**, *96*, 14013–14018. [CrossRef]

medicina

MDPI

Article

Genotyping of Type A Human Respiratory Syncytial Virus Based on Direct F Gene Sequencing

Daifullah Al Aboud [1], Nora M. Al Aboud [2], Mater I. R. Al-Malky [3] and Ahmed S. Abdel-Moneim [1,4,*]

1 College of Medicine, Taif University, Al-Taif 21944, Saudi Arabia; d.alaboud@tu.edu.sa
2 Department of Biology, College of Applied Sciences, Umm Al Qura University, Makkah 21955, Saudi Arabia; nmaboud@uqu.edu.sa
3 Hospital of Paediatrics, Al-Taif 21944, Saudi Arabia; mater1386@hotmail.com
4 Department of Virology, Faculty of Veterinary Medicine, Beni-Suef University, Beni-Suef 62511, Egypt
* Correspondence: asa@bsu.edu.eg or asa@tu.edu.sa

Received: 23 March 2019; Accepted: 14 May 2019; Published: 20 May 2019

Abstract: *Background and objectives:* The human respiratory syncytial virus (hRSV) is among the important respiratory pathogens affecting children. Genotype-specific attachment (G) gene sequencing is usually used to determine the virus genotype. The reliability of the fusion (F) gene vs. G gene genotype-specific sequencing was screened. *Materials and Methods:* Archival RNA from Saudi children who tested positive for hRSV-A were used. Samples were subjected to a conventional one-step RT-PCR for both F and G genes and direct gene sequencing of the amplicons using the same primer sets. Phylogeny and mutational analysis of the obtained sequences were conducted. *Results:* The generic primer set succeeded to amplify target gene sequences. The phylogenetic tree based on partial F gene sequencing resulted in an efficient genotyping of hRSV-A strains equivalent to the partial G gene genotyping method. NA1, ON1, and GA5 genotypes were detected in the clinical samples. The latter was detected for the first time in Saudi Arabia. Different mutations in both conserved and escape-mutant domains were detected in both F and G. *Conclusion:* It was concluded that a partial F gene sequence can be used efficiently for hRSV-A genotyping.

Keywords: hRSV; F gene; G gene; children; respiratory diseases; genotyping; Saudi Arabia

---

1. Introduction

Human respiratory syncytial virus (hRSV) causes considerable respiratory distress with variable severity in infancy and early childhood [1,2]. It is also responsible for the induction of respiratory illness in elderly and immunocompromised patients [3], in addition to being a common nosocomial pathogen [4]. The virus belongs to the family *Pneumoviridae*, genus *Orthopneumovirus*, and possesses a single-stranded negative-sense RNA genome that encodes eleven proteins [5], including both attachment (G) and fusion (F) envelope proteins that work together to attach to the target cell membrane by the G protein [6], while fusion of the viral and cell membranes occurs through the action of the F glycoprotein [7].

The G glycoprotein is a type II surface protein which is highly glycosylated and possesses a considerable degree of nucleotide variability [8]. It possesses two hypervariable regions (HVR1 and HVR2); the HVR2 in the C-terminal region is used to screen the G gene variability of different genotypes [9,10]. Five N-glycosylation sites were detected in HVR2 of the hRSV-A attachment protein [11]. The F protein is more conserved than the G glycoprotein and it is translated as an *F0* precursor that is cleaved twice, resulting in disulfide-linked *F1* (aa 137–574) and *F2* (aa 1–109) subunits along with a short peptide, pep27 (aa 110–136). *F2* possesses heptad repeat C (HRC), while *F1* possesses, at its N terminal, a hydrophobic fusion peptide (FP) followed by two heptad repeats, A and B (HRA and HRB). HRA, HRB, and HRC are essential for envelope fusion to the host cell membrane [12,13]. *F2* possesses five N-glycosylation sites, while HRB, part of *F1*, possesses a single N-glycosylation site; however, *F2* contains more conserved sequence than *F1*, which is characterized by a high homology among different hRSV genotypes [14]. The highly conserved nature of *F2* qualifies it for being a potential target for diagnostic assays.

The hRSV is classified into two major groups: hRSV A and hRSV B [15]. To date, 20 genotypes of hRSV-A and 36 genotypes of hRSV-B are known to exist based on the sequence variation of the G gene [16,17]. Although both hRSV types circulate worldwide, type A was found to be dominant in certain countries [18,19]. Novel genotypes may appear and could replace prevalent genotypes, and many genotypes may circulate together; however, some new genotypes may dominate [20,21]. In 1999, the B/BA genotype, with a duplication of 60 nucleotides of the G gene, appeared [22]; then, the A/ON1 genotype, with a duplication of 72 nucleotides (nt) in the G gene, appeared [23]. Both genotypes are currently prevalent worldwide. The severity of the disease is dependent on the virus genotype, as genotypes A/GA2, A/GA4, A/ON1, and B/BA were found to be of relatively low virulence in comparison to A/NA1, A/GA3, and A/GA5 [24–26].

Typing of hRSV is mainly based on direct G sequencing of sequences flanking HVR2; however, genotype-specific amplification is needed. The F gene could constitute an alternative method for hRSV genotyping; it was found to successfully genotype RSV strains in comparison to the G gene and resulted in the same phylogenetic clusters based on a full genome sequence of the F gene [27]. Accordingly, the aim of the current study was to screen the efficiency of genotyping hRSV-A based on gene sequencing of *F2* and the first part of *F1* (FP and HRA) and compare it with genotype-specific partial G gene sequencing. Genotyping and sequence analysis of the Saudi hRSV-A strains is another objective of the current study.

2. Materials and Methods

2.1. Ethical Statement

Ethical release was obtained from both by the College of Medicine, Taif University (TU/1652/1433/1, approved on 29th April 2011), and also from the hospital of Paediatrics ethical committee based on the human subjects protection guidelines. The first part of the study was previously published [28]. The guardians of the children involved in the study signed informed written consent about the study.

2.2. Samples

A total of 59 archived RNA/DNA samples that showed positive real-time RT-PCR results for hRSV-A, determined in our previous study [28], were used as targets for amplification of F and G genes. The RNA samples were stored at −80 °C. All samples were collected previously from children with respiratory distress from hospital of Paediatrics, Taif, Saudi Arabia, during the period from January to May 2012. The viral load in the samples (n = 56) samples were found to be weak, with a range of 1×10^2 to $1 \times 10^{4.5}$ copies/mL [29].

2.3. One-Step Conventional RT-PCR

An F gene-specific oligonucleotide primer set: Fus-For (1–29) 5′-ATGGAGTTGCCAATCCTCA AAGCAAATGC-3′ and Fus-Rev (622–643) 5′-ATATGCTGCAGCTTTGCTTGTT-3′, that flanks F2 and the first part of F1 (FP and HRA), was designed based on hRSV-A-GZ08-0 (KP218910). G gene genotype-specific primers for ON1/NA1 and GA5 that flank HVR2 in the C-terminal region of the G gene were also designed and used for amplification of the partial G gene based on the result of F gene sequencing. G gene-specific primer sets were as follows: ON1/NA1 (365-384)-For 5′-CTGAGTC AACCCCACAATCC-3′, ON1/NA1-Rev (24–43 G–F intergene UTR) 5′-ATTTGGTCATG GCTTTTTGC-3′ based on based on hRSV-A-GZ08-0 (KP218910) and GA5-For (374–395) 5′-TCCT GCAATCTACAACAGTCAA -3′ and GA5-Rev-(867–889) 5′-CTGTTATGTTGGATGGAGATG-GA-3′

based on RSVA/Homo sapiens/ITA/120/2009 (KF826832) were designed. Reverse transcription was conducted using GoTaq® 1-Step RT-PCR (Promega, Southampton, UK) that was based on GoScript™ Reverse Transcriptase. Briefly, the program was adjusted for reverse transcription at 45 °C for 45 min, followed by an initial denaturation step at 95 °C for 5 min and 35 cycles of 95 °C for 30 s, 50 °C for 30 s, and 72 °C for 1 min. This was followed by a final 10 min elongation step at 72 °C. The RT-PCR amplicons were subjected to 1.5% agarose gel electrophoresis.

2.4. Direct Sequencing and Gene Sequence Analysis

Amplicons with the expected size were excised from the gel and then purified using a gel-extraction kit (Koma Biotek, Seoul, Korea). The purified amplicons were used as templates for direct sequencing using the same primers as those used for the F and G genes' amplification. Sequencing was performed commercially using the BigDye v.3.1 Applied Biosystems (Foster City, CA, USA) kit according to the manufacturer's protocol. Raw sequences were visualized and analyzed using MEGA 5.2. Homology BLASTn searches from different strains were performed using highly similar sequences (megablast) against published hRSV sequences in the GenBank databases using default algorithm parameters. The gene sequences of both F and G genes were deposited in GenBank under the accession numbers: F (KU924011-KU924023) and G (MK182708-MK182720). CLUSTAL W multisequence analysis was performed and the phylogenetic tree was constructed using the maximum likelihood statistical method with 1000 bootstrap replicates and Tamura–Nei model substitution model. Nucleotide variability among different strains was calculated using the CLUSTALW available in GenomeNet Database [30].

2.5. Deduced Amino Acid Sequence and Sequence Analysis

Deduced amino acid sequences of both F and G amino acid sequences were compared using MEGA 5.2. Amino acid substitutions at different functional and structural protein fragments were analysed. The polyphen (polymorphism phenotyping) prediction webtool [31] was used to screen the potential effect of amino acid substitutions among strains on the function.

3. Results

3.1. Direct Sequencing and Phylogenetic Analysis

Both generic primers for F and G genes were successful in amplification of the strains, showing relatively high viral load for 13 of the 59 samples (≥1 × $10^{3.5}$ copies/mL). The F gene domains of the hRSV-A isolates possess about 10% nucleotide variability. The signal peptide, however, showed higher nucleotide variability. Partial F gene sequencing revealed that the Saudi strains in the current study belong to the NA1 genotype (6/13, 46.15%), ON1 (5/13; 38.46%), and GA5 genotype (2/13; 15.38%) (Figure 1a). Partial G gene sequencing using strain-specific primers for these strains confirmed the correct strain classification obtained by using F gene sequencing, and similar clustering of the hRSV strains was obtained using both genes (Figure 1a,b). The F gene domains of the hRSV-A isolates possess about 10% nucleotide variability. The signal peptide and transmembrane domains, however, showed nucleotide variability to be higher than detected in the HVRs of the G gene (data not shown).

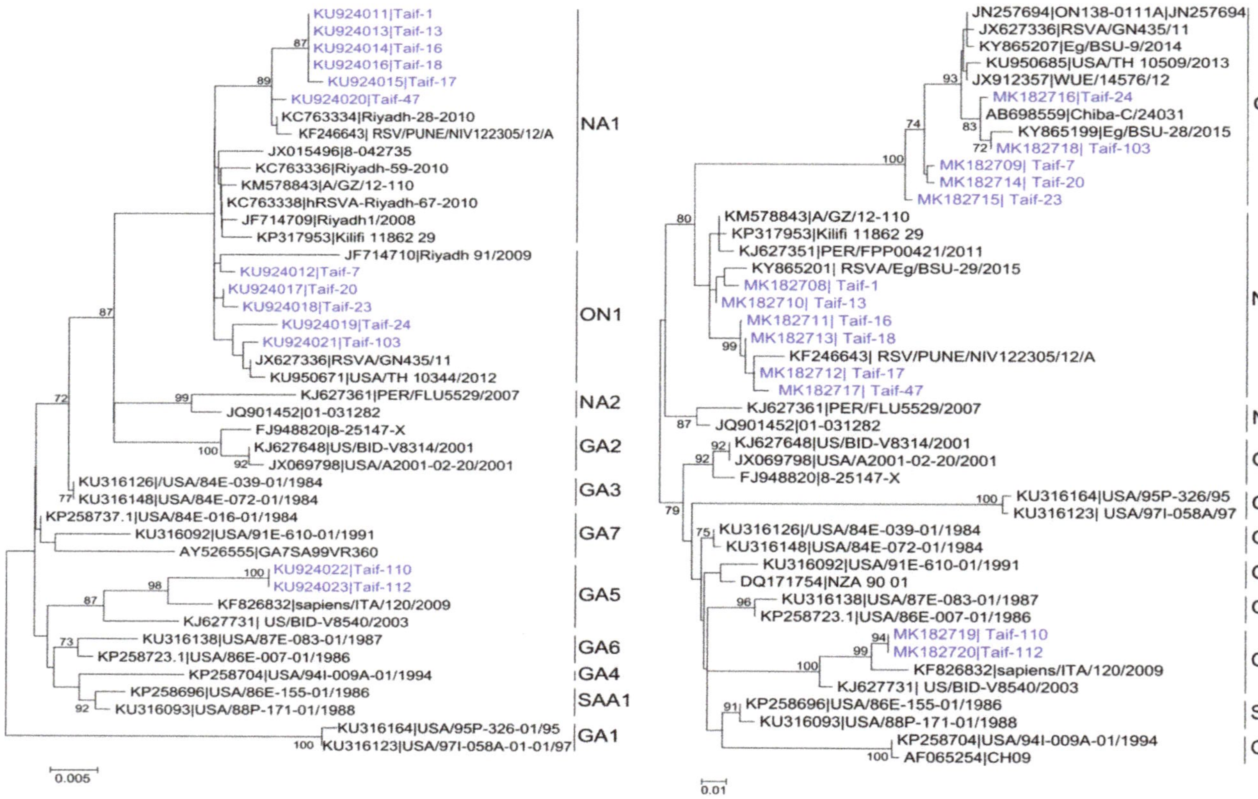

Figure 1. Phylogenetic trees of the nucleotide sequences of partial fusion (F) and attachment (G) genes of human respiratory syncytial virus A (hRSV-A) strains from Saudi Arabia in comparison to relevant published strains. (**a**) F gene; (**b**) G gene. The maximum likelihood tree was constructed using MEGA 5.2 freeware. Strains detected in the current study are shown in blue color. Only bootstrap values above 70% are shown.

3.2. *Deduced Amino Acid Sequence and Sequence Analysis*

Five N-glycosylation sites, N27, N70, N116, N120, and N126, were found to be conserved among all the thirteen Saudi strains, except for strain Taif-103, that has lost one of the N-glycosylations at N120 (Figure 2). The fusion protein of Taif-20, Taif-23, Taif-110, and Taif-112 showed S-to-N substitution at position 105 just before the first cleavage (Figure 2), with no potential effect on the function as demonstrated by the polymorphism phenotyping prediction tool (data not shown). Seven amino acid substitutions—L3F, T11I, I19T, T13A, L15F, A16T, and I19T—were detected in the signal peptide, and three—T120A, T125N, and V127I—amino acid substitutions were detected in the p27 domain (Figure 2).

A duplication of amino acids (QEETLHSTTSEGYLSPSQVYTTS) was found in two regions within the G protein which reflects an 72 nt insert characteristic to the ON1 genotype (Figure 3). L298P, V303A, and Y304H amino acid substitutions were detected in all ON1 Saudi strains, Y273N was detected in Taif 23, and L274P was detected in Taif-24 and Taif-103 strains (Figure 3). The P310L substitution, equivalent to P286L in viruses that have no duplication, was recorded in 10 out of the 13 Saudi strains. There is an existence of accumulated signature coding changes in the epitope regions of the G protein (Figure 3). Variations among the N-glycosylation site of HVR2 of the Saudi strains' attachment proteins were detected. Interestingly, all Saudi NA1 and ON1 strains except Taif-24 and Taif-103 showed N237D amino acid substitution that resulted in loss of the N237 N-glycosylation site. N250 was found only in Saudi GA5 strains, while N251 was detected in 2/5 ON1 and 6/6 of the NA1 Saudi strains. N273 was detected only in Saudi GA5 strains, as well as a single ON1 Saudi strain. N294 (N318 in ON1 genotypes) was detected in the majority of Saudi ON1 and NA1 strains, but none of the Saudi GA5 strains or the A2 prototype strain (Figure 3).

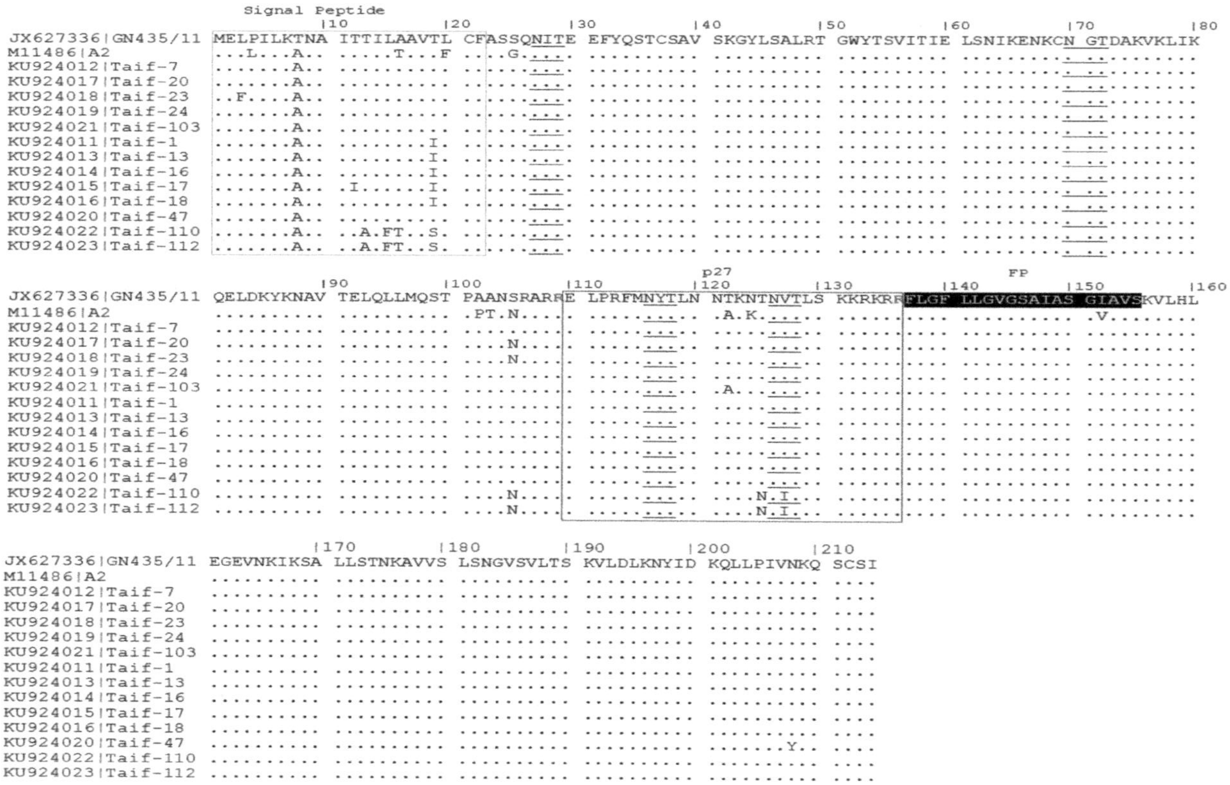

Figure 2. Deduced amino acid sequences of partial fusion proteins from different Saudi hRSV-A strains. Highlighted are the signal peptide (1–22) (blue box), heptad repeat domain C (75–97), cleavage site-1 (CS-1) and cleavage site-2 (CS-2) at Arg109 (NSRARR↓E) and Arg136 (KKRKRR↓F) (red color), p27 (110–136) (green box), fusion peptide (FP) (137–155), and heptad repeat domain A (153–end of the current sequence). The N-glycosylation sites, NXT/S, where X is not a proline, are underlined.

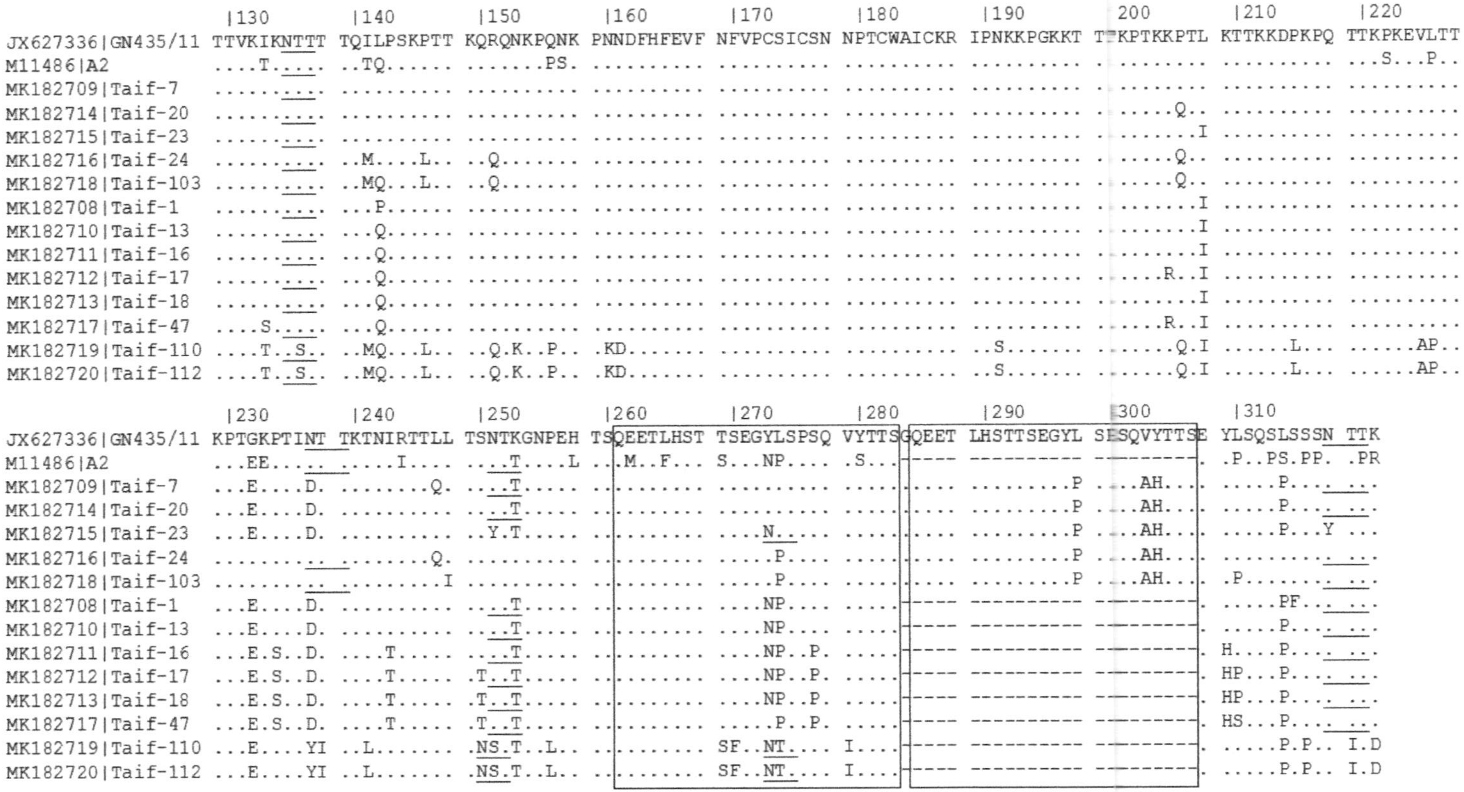

Figure 3. Deduced amino acid sequences of the partial attachment protein (G) from different Saudi hRSV-A strains. The N-glycosylation sites, NXT/S, where X is not a proline, are underlined. Duplicated regions in the ON1 strains are shown in the boxes.

4. Discussion

Both of the designed generic primers were successful in amplification of the three different genotypes of hRSV-A, ON1, NA1, and GA5, that were detected among Saudi archival RNA samples. It is also assumed that the generic F primer set could detect all hRSV-A strains, since it showed complete identities to most of the published hRSV-A strains except for a single mismatch detected occasionally. Genotyping based on partial gene sequencing of both F and G genes showed similar results, which denotes that the designed F gene could be used efficiently in genotyping of hRSV-A strains.

The Saudi strains in the current study are classified as NA1, ON1, and GA5 genotypes. Both NA1 and GA5 showed higher virulence to the children in comparison to ON1 and other hRSV-A strains [24–26]. Two out of the thirteen strains were related to GA5, and this represents the first record of this subtype in Saudi Arabia. In Saudi Arabia, only a few studies have been conducted on hRSV genotypes; however, the hRSV-A type, mostly the NA-1 subtype, is the dominant genotype [32,33]. The hRSV-A ON1 genotype was detected for the first time in Canada in 2010 [23]. A Saudi strain in the GenBank database was found to be closely related to the ON1 strain isolated in 2009 in Riyadh and also closely related to ON1 strains detected in the current study from Al-Taif. This finding reveals that the ON1 strains have circulated in Saudi Arabia since 2009. This assumption is confirmed by the global data that suggested that the ancestor of ON1 emerged during 2008–2009 [34].

It is known that the F protein is focused on the signal peptide, p27, transmembrane domain, and ø antigenic site [35]. Similarly, the highest variability among amino acids among Saudi strains was detected in the signal peptide, followed by the p27 domain of the fusion protein. The fusion protein of hRSV strain harbors six N-glycosylation sites [9,36], which were confirmed to be conserved among the current Saudi strains, except for strain Taif-103 (A/ON1), which has lost one of the N-glycosylations at N120. It is known that N-glycosylation is important for the folding and transport of viral proteins and hence virus infectivity [37]. It is worth mentioning here that the three N-glycosylation sites—N116, N120, and N126—are found in close proximity to the proteolytic cleavage site [38,39]. It seems that the T122A amino acid substitution that resulted in a loss of the N-glycosylation site in Taif-103 does not affect the fusion or the proteolytic affinity of the protein, as confirmed previously [38].

The deduced amino acid sequence of the G gene revealed the presence of L298P, V303A, and Y304H amino acid substitution in all ON1 Saudi strains. Y273N was detected in Taif 23 and L274P was detected in the Taif-24 and Taif-103 strains. Such substitutions are considered noteworthy as they are present next to aa 265–273 (antigenic site) [40]. The P310L was recorded in the majority of the Saudi strains. Positively selected residues reported by Botosso et al., were found to be conserved in the Saudi ON1 and NA1 strains, except at the residues T237D and L274P [41] that constituted escape-mutant screened monoclonal antibodies [42,43]. The N273 N-glycosylation site was lost in the Saudi NA1 and most of the ON1 strains, which was also observed in NA1 strains from Japan and China [11,20]. Absence of the N250 site in all Saudi strains except for Saudi GA5 strains was expected, since it is a specific N-glycosylation site for both GA5 and SAA1 of hRSV-A [11]. The variation of the number of N-glycosylation sites was found to be associated with altered antigenicity [44].

5. Conclusions

Direct partial F gene sequencing represents an accurate method for hRSV-A genotyping that matched partial G gene sequencing results. The current study provides evidence of the circulation of GA5, NA1, and ON1 genotypes in Saudi Arabia. Although mutations in conserved or escape-mutant domains were detected in both F and G proteins, most of them do not affect the virus' virulence.

Author Contributions: D.A.A., N.M.A.A., and A.S.A.-M. designed the primers, conducted the RT-PCR, and analyzed the sequences. M.I.R.A.-M. and A.S.A.-M. conceived the study design. D.A.A. and N.M.A.A. drafted the manuscript. A.S.A.-M. and M.I.R.A.-M. critically revised the manuscript.

Funding: This research received no external funding.

Conflicts of Interest: The authors have no conflicts of interest to declare.

References

1. Nair, H.; Nokes, D.J.; Gessner, B.D.; Dherani, M.; Madhi, S.A.; Singleton, R.J.; O'Brien, K.L.; Roca, A.; Wright, P.F.; Bruce, N.; et al. Global burden of acute lower respiratory infections due to respiratory syncytial virus in young children: A systematic review and meta-analysis. *Lancet* **2010**, *375*, 1545–1555. [CrossRef]
2. Weber, M.W.; Mulholland, E.K.; Greenwood, B.M. Respiratory syncytial virus infection in tropical and developing countries. *Trop. Med. Int. Health* **1998**, *3*, 268–280. [PubMed]
3. Falsey, A.R.; Hennessey, P.A.; Formica, M.A.; Cox, C.; Walsh, E.E. Respiratory syncytial virus infection in elderly and high-risk adults. *N. Engl. J. Med.* **2005**, *352*, 1749–1759. [CrossRef] [PubMed]
4. French, C.E.; McKenzie, B.C.; Coope, C.; Rajanaidu, S.; Paranthaman, K.; Pebody, R.; Nguyen-Van-Tam, J.S.; Noso-RSV Study Group; Higgins, J.P.; Beck, C.R. Risk of nosocomial respiratory syncytial virus infection and effectiveness of control measures to prevent transmission events: A systematic review. *Influ. Resp. Virus.* **2016**, *10*, 268–290. [CrossRef] [PubMed]
5. Collins, P.L.; Melero, J.A. Progress in understanding and controlling respiratory syncytial virus: Still crazy after all these years. *Virus Res.* **2011**, *162*, 80–99. [CrossRef] [PubMed]
6. Levine, S.; Klaiber-Franco, R.; Paradiso, P.R. Demonstration that glycoprotein G is the attachment protein of respiratory syncytial virus. *J. Gen. Virol.* **1987**, *68*, 2521–2524. [CrossRef] [PubMed]
7. Walsh, E.E.; Hruska, J. Monoclonal antibodies to respiratory syncytial virus proteins: Identification of the fusion protein. *J. Virol.* **1983**, *47*, 171–177. [PubMed]
8. Wertz, G.W.; Krieger, M.; Ball, L.A. Structure and cell surface maturation of the attachment glycoprotein of human respiratory syncytial virus in a cell line deficient in O glycosylation. *J. Virol.* **1989**, *63*, 4767–4776. [PubMed]
9. Melero, J.A. Molecular biology of human respiratory syncytial virus. *Persp. Med. Virol.* **2007**, *14*, 1–42.
10. Melero, J.A.; Mas, V.; McLellan, J.S. Structural, antigenic and immunogenic features of respiratory syncytial virus glycoproteins relevant for vaccine development. *Vaccine* **2017**, *35*, 461–468. [CrossRef] [PubMed]
11. Cui, G.; Zhu, R.; Qian, Y.; Deng, J.; Zhao, L.; Sun, Y.; Wang, F. Genetic variation in attachment glycoprotein genes of human respiratory syncytial virus subgroups a and B in children in recent five consecutive years. *PLoS ONE* **2013**, *8*, e75020-e. [CrossRef]
12. Bermingham, I.M.; Chappell, K.J.; Watterson, D.; Young, P.R. The heptad repeat C domain of the respiratory syncytial virus fusion protein plays a key role in membrane fusion. *J. Virol.* **2018**, *92*, e01323-17. [CrossRef] [PubMed]
13. Zhao, X.; Singh, M.; Malashkevich, V.N.; Kim, P.S. Structural characterization of the human respiratory syncytial virus fusion protein core. *Proc. Natl. Acad. Sci. USA* **2000**, *97*, 14172–14177. [CrossRef] [PubMed]
14. Lopez, J.A.; Bustos, R.; Orvell, C.; Berois, M.; Arbiza, J.; Garcia-Barreno, B.; Melero, J.A. Antigenic structure of human respiratory syncytial virus fusion glycoprotein. *J. Virol.* **1998**, *72*, 6922–6928. [PubMed]
15. Anderson, L.J.; Hierholzer, J.C.; Tsou, C.; Hendry, R.M.; Fernie, B.F.; Stone, Y.; McIntosh, K. Antigenic characterization of respiratory syncytial virus strains with monoclonal antibodies. *J. Infect. Dis.* **1985**, *151*, 626–633. [CrossRef]
16. Malekshahi, S.S.; Razaghipour, S.; Samieipoor, Y.; Hashemi, F.B.; Manesh, A.A.R.; Izadi, A.; Faghihloo, E.; Ghavami, N.; Mokhtari-Azad, T.; Salimi, V. Molecular characterization of the glycoprotein and fusion protein in human respiratory syncytial virus subgroup A: Emergence of ON-1 genotype in Iran. *Infect. Genet. Evol.* **2019**, *71*, 166–178. [CrossRef] [PubMed]
17. Gaymard, A.; Bouscambert-Duchamp, M.; Pichon, M.; Frobert, E.; Vallee, J.; Lina, B.; Casalegno, J.S.; Morfin, F. Genetic characterization of respiratory syncytial virus highlights a new BA genotype and emergence of the ON1 genotype in Lyon, France, between 2010 and 2014. *J. Clin. Virol.* **2018**, *102*, 12–18. [CrossRef] [PubMed]
18. Meng, J.; Stobart, C.C.; Hotard, A.L.; Moore, M.L. An overview of respiratory syncytial virus. *PLoS Pathog.* **2014**, *10*, e1004016. [CrossRef] [PubMed]
19. Pankovics, P.; Szabo, H.; Szekely, G.; Gyurkovits, K.; Reuter, G. Detection and molecular epidemiology of respiratory syncytial virus type A and B strains in childhood respiratory infections in Hungary. *Orvosi Hetilap* **2009**, *150*, 121–127. [CrossRef]
20. Shobugawa, Y.; Saito, R.; Sano, Y.; Zaraket, H.; Suzuki, Y.; Kumaki, A.; Dapat, I.; Oguma, T.; Yamaguchi, M.; Suzuki, H. Emerging genotypes of human respiratory syncytial virus subgroup A among patients in Japan. *J. Clin. Microbiol.* **2009**, *47*, 2475–2482. [CrossRef] [PubMed]

21. Katzov-Eckert, H.; Botosso, V.F.; Neto, E.A.; Zanotto, P.M. Phylodynamics and dispersal of HRSV entails its permanence in the general population in between yearly outbreaks in children. *PLoS ONE* **2012**, *7*, e41953. [CrossRef] [PubMed]
22. Trento, A.; Galiano, M.; Videla, C.; Carballal, G.; Garcia-Barreno, B.; Melero, J.A.; Palomo, C. Major changes in the G protein of human respiratory syncytial virus isolates introduced by a duplication of 60 nucleotides. *J. Gen. Virol.* **2003**, *84*, 3115–3120. [CrossRef] [PubMed]
23. Eshaghi, A.; Duvvuri, V.R.; Lai, R.; Nadarajah, J.T.; Li, A.; Patel, S.N.; Low, D.E.; Gubbay, J.B. Genetic variability of human respiratory syncytial virus A strains circulating in Ontario: A novel genotype with a 72 nucleotide G gene duplication. *PLoS ONE* **2012**, *7*, e32807. [CrossRef] [PubMed]
24. Midulla, F.; Nenna, R.; Scagnolari, C.; Petrarca, L.; Frassanito, A.; Viscido, A.; Arima, S.; Antonelli, G.; Pierangeli, A. How respiratory syncytial virus genotypes influence the clinical course in infants hospitalized for bronchiolitis. *J. Infect. Dis.* **2019**, *219*, 526–534. [CrossRef] [PubMed]
25. Rodriguez-Fernandez, R.; Tapia, L.I.; Yang, C.F.; Torres, J.P.; Chavez-Bueno, S.; Garcia, C.; Jaramillo, L.M.; Moore-Clingenpeel, M.; Jafri, H.S.; Peeples, M.E.; et al. Respiratory syncytial virus genotypes, host immune profiles, and disease severity in young children hospitalized with bronchiolitis. *J. Infect. Dis.* **2017**, *217*, 24–34. [CrossRef]
26. Martinello, R.A.; Chen, M.D.; Weibel, C.; Kahn, J.S. Correlation between respiratory syncytial virus genotype and severity of illness. *J. Infect. Dis.* **2002**, *186*, 839–842. [CrossRef] [PubMed]
27. Song, J.; Wang, H.; Ng, T.I.; Cui, A.; Zhu, S.; Huang, Y.; Sun, L.; Yang, Z.; Yu, D.; Yu, P.; et al. Sequence analysis of the fusion protein gene of human respiratory syncytial virus circulating in China from 2003 to 2014. *Sci. Rep.* **2018**, *8*, 17618. [CrossRef]
28. Abdel-Moneim, A.S.; Kamel, M.M.; Al-Ghamdi, A.S.; Al-Malky, M.I. Detection of bocavirus in children suffering from acute respiratory tract infections in Saudi Arabia. *PLoS ONE* **2013**, *8*, e55500. [CrossRef]
29. Abdel-Moneim, A.S.; Shehab, G.M.; Alsulaimani, A.A.; Al-Malky, M.I.R. Development of TaqMan RT-qPCR for the detection of type A human respiratory syncytial virus. *Mol. Cell. Probes* **2017**, *33*, 16–19. [CrossRef] [PubMed]
30. GenomeNet. Available online: https://www.genome.jp (accessed on 24 May 2019).
31. PolyPhen-2 (Polymorphism Phenotyping v2). Available online: http://genetics.bwh.harvard.edu/pph2/ (accessed on 10 October 2017).
32. Almajhdi, F.N.; Farrag, M.A.; Amer, H.M. Genetic diversity in the G protein gene of group A human respiratory syncytial viruses circulating in Riyadh, Saudi Arabia. *Arch. Virol.* **2014**, *159*, 73–81. [CrossRef] [PubMed]
33. AlMajhdi, F.N.; Al-Jarallah, A.; Elaeed, M.; Latif, A.; Gissmann, L.; Amer, H.M. Prevalence of respiratory syncytial virus infection in Riyadh during the winter season 2007–2008 and different risk factors impact. *Int. J. Virol.* **2009**, *5*, 154–163.
34. Duvvuri, V.R.; Granados, A.; Rosenfeld, P.; Bahl, J.; Eshaghi, A.; Gubbay, J.B. Genetic diversity and evolutionary insights of respiratory syncytial virus A ON1 genotype: Global and local transmission dynamics. *Sci. Rep.* **2015**, *5*, 14268. [CrossRef] [PubMed]
35. Hause, A.M.; Henke, D.M.; Avadhanula, V.; Shaw, C.A.; Tapia, L.I.; Piedra, P.A. Sequence variability of the respiratory syncytial virus (RSV) fusion gene among contemporary and historical genotypes of RSV/A and RSV/B. *PLoS ONE* **2017**, *12*, e0175792-e.
36. Kornfeld, R.; Kornfeld, S. Assembly of asparagine-linked oligosaccharides. *Ann. Rev. Biochem.* **1985**, *54*, 631–664. [CrossRef]
37. Bieberich, E. Synthesis, processing, and function of N-glycans in N-glycoproteins. *Adv. Neurobiol.* **2014**, *9*, 47–70. [PubMed]
38. Zimmer, G.; Trotz, I.; Herrler, G. N-glycans of F protein differentially affect fusion activity of human respiratory syncytial virus. *J. Virol.* **2001**, *75*, 4744–4751. [CrossRef] [PubMed]
39. Lambert, D.M. Role of oligosaccharides in the structure and function of respiratory syncytial virus glycoproteins. *Virology* **1988**, *164*, 458–466. [CrossRef]
40. Cane, P. Molecular Epidemiology and Evolution of RSV. In *Respiratory Syncytial Virus*; Elsevier: Amsterdam, The Netherlands, 2007; pp. 89–113.

41. Botosso, V.F.; Zanotto, P.M.; Ueda, M.; Arruda, E.; Gilio, A.E.; Vieira, S.E.; Stewien, K.E.; Peret, T.C.; Jamal, L.F.; Pardini, M.I.; et al. Positive selection results in frequent reversible amino acid replacements in the G protein gene of human respiratory syncytial virus. *PLoS Pathog.* **2009**, *5*, e1000254. [CrossRef] [PubMed]
42. Garcia, O.; Martin, M.; Dopazo, J.; Arbiza, J.; Frabasile, S.; Russi, J.; Hortal, M.; Perez-Breña, P.; Martínez, I.; García-Barreno, B.; et al. Evolutionary pattern of human respiratory syncytial virus (subgroup A): Cocirculating lineages and correlation of genetic and antigenic changes in the G glycoprotein. *J. Virol.* **1994**, *68*, 5448–5459.
43. Martinez, I.; Dopazo, J.; Melero, J.A. Antigenic structure of the human respiratory syncytial virus G glycoprotein and relevance of hypermutation events for the generation of antigenic variants. *J. Gen. Virol.* **1997**, *78*, 2419–2429. [CrossRef]
44. Palomo, C.; Cane, P.A.; Melero, J.A. Evaluation of the antibody specificities of human convalescent-phase sera against the attachment (G) protein of human respiratory syncytial virus: Influence of strain variation and carbohydrate side chains. *J. Med. Virol.* **2000**, *60*, 468–474. [CrossRef]

MDPI
St. Alban-Anlage 66
4052 Basel
Switzerland
Tel. +41 61 683 77 34
Fax +41 61 302 89 18
www.mdpi.com

Medicina Editorial Office
E-mail: medicina@mdpi.com
www.mdpi.com/journal/medicina

www.ingramcontent.com/pod-product-compliance
Lightning Source LLC
LaVergne TN
LVHW070541100526
838202LV00012B/340